HANDBOOK OF
BLOOD PRESSURE MONITORING

John M. R. Bruner, MD
Massachusetts General Hospital
and
Harvard Medical School

PSG Publishing Company, Inc.
Littleton, Massachusetts

Library of Congress Cataloging in Publication Data

Bruner, John M R   1925-
  Blood pressure monitoring.

  (Postgraduate clinical techniques series; v. 1)
  Bibliography: p.
  Includes index.
  1. Blood pressure—Measurement. I. Title.
II. Series. [DNLM: 1. Blood pressure determination—
Methods—Handbooks. 2. Monitoring, Physiologic—Methods
—Handbooks. WG106 B894h]
QP105.2.B78   612'.14   78-16876
ISBN 0-88416-228-1

Printed in the United States of America.

International Standard Book Number: 0-88416-228-1

Library of Congress Catalog Card Number: 78-16876

lev
11-13-80

CONTENTS

INTRODUCTION

In an attempt to maintain cerebral perfusion by "keeping the blood pressure up," a neurosurgical patient is given an infusion of a vasopressor. As the blood pressure is checked by several different methods of measurement, consternation is expressed over the wide disparity in values obtained. The radial artery pressure shown on an oscilloscope is 210 mm Hg systolic, 60 mm Hg diastolic; but when a pressure cuff on the same arm is slowly deflated, deflections do not appear on the oscilloscope until the cuff pressure has declined to 100 mm Hg. By auscultation it is very difficult to determine the patient's blood pressure at all; only a few faint sounds are heard at 90 mm Hg.

Is the monitor "wrong"? What is the "right" blood pressure? Why are there such large and distressing discrepancies between blood pressure values obtained by different methods?

A complex series of events determines blood pressure. Included are not only the contractile function of the ventricle, the filling of the arterial tree, and "runoff" through peripheral resistance, but also reflections of energy and the effects of resonance in the vascular tree and in external coupling and obervation systems. Any single method of measuring this "pressure" merely looks at a particular selection of artifacts. Utilizing the Riva-Rocci method, one listens for sounds of turbulence generated by flow in a partially compressed vessel. Doppler techniques look at vessel wall motion or axial flow. Still another blood pressure device, the oscillotonometer, is a mechanically amplified plethysmograph. The "occlusion technique" combines a proximal cuff with an indwelling arterial cannula. This method is often intuitively assumed to be "right," but commonly gives systolic values quite at variance from peak systolic excursions of the directly measured pressure pulse as displayed on the cathode ray tube.

Since one is looking at different things through different measurement techniques, should it really come as a surprise that the observed numbers are different? Blood pressure depends in large part on the circumstances of measurement.

The purpose of this text is to provide an understanding of pulsatile pressure and its measurement in order that the clinician may better select and measure those pressure phenomena that promise to contain information pertinent to the care of his patients.

i

Without defining what is the "right" measurement technique, the intent is to facilitate acquisition of useful information from existing observation methods and to enhance confidence in the equipment at hand. For the serious clinical investigator using invasive techniques, I point to a special obligation: he should be aware that it is appropriate to compare numbers and wave forms from different systems only if the fidelity of each system is known and preferably identical. A significant portion of the numbers and wave forms observed with invasive techniques may, in fact, be generated by the monitoring system itself.

This text presents an analysis of the elements of the systemic arterial pressure pulse. That analysis will then be related to techniques of measurement and to clinical applications of those techniques. Passing reference is made to venous pressure and pulmonary vascular pressure only as concepts; techniques and problems pertinent to the main theme of the text are also applicable to measurement of low pressures. Interpretations of venous and pulmonary pressure are fields unto themselves and will not be treated here.

Texts and articles exist in abundance on the measurement of blood pressure. What is different about this presentation is that it is written for clinicians—technicians, nurses, and physicians responsible for hour-to-hour care of the critically ill. Clinical personnel have demands on their time that preclude acquiring and maintaining familiarity with advanced physics and mathematics, the esoterica of which have little perceptible clinical applicability. Therefore, my aim is to develop a sense of familiarity with concepts that have clear clinical pertinence, and do this through example and analogy while eschewing all but the simplest mathematics.

To this end deliberate digressions in style and subject matter characterize the first two chapters. Chapter 1, Fundamentals, establishes general concepts and a common language. Offering a variety of examples, purposely redundant, occasionally arch, the chapter is akin to a series of five-finger exercises serving to promote agility in the appreciation of dynamic phenomena. While drawn from nature and familiar mechanics, the examples and analogies embody truths that are directly transferable to human physiology and clinical technology.

Chapter 2, Considerations in the Design of a Pumping System, is presented in the belief that one can be more sympathetic to the operational complexities and vagaries of a system if there is understanding of the objectives and the design constraints that prevailed during evolution of the mechanism.

No pretenses are offered as to comprehensive coverage or evenness of presentation. Some topics have been slighted, usually owing to lack of firsthand experience; others have been treated elaborately, even repetitiously, because they interested me, may or should interest others, deserved emphasis, or have been observed as loci of concern or error. Since no adequate description of the oscillotonometer could be found in the literature, it was necessary to write one for Chapter 4. The shift register display is treated at length because it augers to be *the* display mode from this point on; those who use or buy such equipment ought to have some idea of how it works and what it does.

The sermon on Monitors, Science, Commerce, and Regulation in Chapter 5 is based on a decade of observing that the worship of procedures and equipment not only tends to divert attention from intelligent care of patients, but also enables the icon vendors, temple builders, and administrative priesthood to filch ever larger fractions of the health care dollar.

Avoidance of speculation and editorial bias have not been among my goals.

John M. R. Bruner

1 Fundamentals: Waves, Horns, Estuaries, and Weighty Words

When you can measure what you are speaking about, and express it in numbers, you know something about it; but when you cannot measure it, cannot express it in numbers, your knowledge is of a meagre and unsatisfactory kind; it may be the beginning of knowledge, but you have scarcely, in your thoughts, advanced to the stage of *science,* whatever the matter may be.

Attributed to Lord Kelvin.

1

I believe that I can understand a process only when I can construct some sort of a visual image of just how it operates.

John W. Remington[56]

PRESSURE

Pressure is force per unit area. Force is measured in dynes; area, in square centimeters. But we use a measure of *length*—millimeters (of mercury)—to characterize pressure. Why? The answer lies in man's proclivity to describe and calibrate phenomena with reference to tools that happen to be available. The exercise is continued as long as it proves expedient and reliable. Measurement of blood pressure was first accomplished by observing how high a column of blood would rise in a tube attached to the artery in a horse's neck. Later, manometers filled with mercury proved more convenient. The height of a fluid column can be used as an indicator of pressure because the force of gravity is constant over the surface of the earth. One does not have to carry around a calibrated spring. Anyone with a fluid-filled tube of any diameter or shape can make reproducible pressure measurements that are comparable to measurements made elsewhere on the face of the planet.

All bets are off if one is in space or subject to the gravitational force of a different celestial body. In recognition of this a general unit for pressure was established: "torr," after the Italian physicist Torricelli. On the earth one torr is the same as one millimeter of mercury.

If work* and resistance are to be computed from physiologic pressure measurements, then it becomes necessary to convert familiar manometric pressure into compatible units. This accounts for the peculiar factors that appear in standard equations.

---

*Work is force times distance. The units are dynes and centimeters; the product, work, is measured in dyne-cm.

Pertinent formulas are these:

(1) vascular resistance =

$$\frac{\text{pressure difference in mm Hg}}{\text{flow in liters/minute}} \quad \text{x } 80 =$$

resistance in dyne-sec-cm^{-5}.

This is based on the fact that

(2) $P = 0.1 \cdot g \cdot \varrho Hg \cdot h$

or

(3) $P = 1323$ x mm Hg

where

P = pressure in dynes/cm^2
g = acceleration of gravity in cm/sec^2
ϱHg = "rho" Hg = density of Hg in gm/cm^3
h = height of column of Hg in mm

To confound the issue further, another unit of pressure will be encountered in the International System (SI). Here the unit for pressure is the pascal, equal to 10 dynes/cm^2.

Pressure does not exist as an isolated value. Pressure is a relationship: the differential force (per unit area) between two specified points or "across" a component of the system. When looking at the pressure drop across a vascular resistance such as that of the lung, one measures the upstream pressure (relative to atmospheric), the downstream pressure (again relative to atmospheric), and subtracts the latter from the former. This, then, is the pressure drop across the vascular resistance.

While the zero reference point for physiologic pressure measurement is atmospheric pressure, there may be no observable points in a complex physiologic hydraulic system that are actually at "zero" pressure; some points may even be subatmospheric.

Any given point may have several pressure relationships. The diastolic filling pressure of the left ventricle, for example, may have one value relative to atmospheric, but quite a different value relative to intrapericardial pressure.

WAVES

A wave is a traveling disturbance that carries energy. The medium through which the wave moves is disturbed but the medium does not travel with the wave. Indeed, the medium may have both velocity and direction quite different from that of the wave. Consider this example: a cork bobs on the surface of a slowly undulating ocean as the waves pass by. When viewed at a right angle to the direction of travel of the ocean wave, the motion of the cork is circular: upward and in the direction of wave's travel as the crest passes, then down and backward into the trough. But the cork, like the molecules of water in the wave, does not travel. Indeed, a cork floating in the Gulf Stream may be moving northeasterly while the wind is generating waves that move in a southwesterly direction. Consider also a storm: lightning generates thunder claps that travel through the air at the speed of sound. If you, the observer, are standing south of the storm, the wind may be blowing 40 miles per hour northward into the center of the storm, while the sound of the thunder travels to you at 600 miles per hour in the opposite, southerly direction. Thus the direction of *flow* of the medium is not necessarily related to the direction of wave travel through it.

Waves are characterized by *frequency,* by intensity or *amplitude,* * by direction, and by *velocity.* The *frequency* of a wave is the number of crests passing in a given unit of time. The *period* of a wave is the time interval between each wave crest and is the reciprocal of frequency. The frequency of waves is usually expressed in hertz (abbreviation: Hz). One hertz is equal to one wave cycle per second. *Wave length* is the distance between wave crests. The relationship between period and wave length is established by the velocity at which the wave travels through a specific medium. For each type of wave disturbance (for example, sound or light) there is a fixed velocity in a given medium (water, air). The intensity or *amplitude* of a wave is a measure of the perturbation of the medium from its resting state. In the case of a water wave, the amplitude is

---

*Strictly speaking, intensity is related to the square of the amplitude.

half the vertical distance from the crest of the wave to the next succeeding trough. (Here one again sees how "pressure," measured as the height of a medium, becomes involved with amplitude in the case of fluid waves.)

Complex Waves and Fundamentals

> The decomposition of pulsatile signals into sinusoidal components is always (mathematically) possible, provided certain conditions are fulfilled....Whether or not one gains insight into the system studied by this is a different question...
>
> U. Gessner[24]

All waves that occur in nature can be described as sine waves. Their contour is that of the graph of the sine of an angle plotted against degrees of rotation as the angle is rotated through 360°. In complex waves, disturbances having different frequencies are superimposed one upon the other. No matter how complex the wave, however, it may be regarded as the sum or composite of a fundamental frequency plus a number of harmonic frequencies. Harmonics are integral multiples of the fundamental frequency.

Wave Qualities, Square and Otherwise

When the amplitude of a sine wave is plotted against time (or degrees of rotation), the plot describes an almost straight line as it passes through the x axis at zero amplitude. The slope of the line at the "zero crossing" becomes more vertical under either of two conditions: (1) When the peak amplitude or intensity of the wave is increased, or (2) if frequency is increased. Each condition is said to increase the "steepness" of a "wave front" (a wave disturbance starting anew from zero amplitude).

The steepness or rate of rise of a wave front is called (perhaps inaccurately) "slew rate."[36] This parameter is of concern in certain signal processing problems: in the design of ECG monitors to reject pacemaker artifacts, or in enabling a demand pacemaker to discriminate between an R wave and a tall T wave.

One criterion of the quality of a recording system is its ability to handle steep wave fronts or "transients." The ultimate of steep

6

wave fronts is a "step function:" a change in amplitude occurring instantaneously. A "square wave" is a double step function, akin to turning a switch on, then off again. It is a very stressful signal. A great deal of information can be inferred from the manner in which a system under test handles a square wave. If the system can lag, rattle, or fade, it will do so! In Figure 1-1, A is a square wave slightly distorted by somewhat limited low frequency response in the recorder. In Figure 1-1, panel H, the rounded upstroke indicates poor response to high frequency. In Figure 1-2 "ringing" or spurious oscillation indicates that the system is significantly underdamped.* In Figure 1-1, panels B, C, and D, system output falls off with passage of time, an indication of limited response to low frequency.

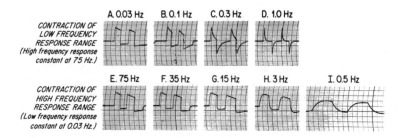

Figure 1-1 Recording System Response to Square Wave Input In each panel two square waves have been applied to the input of a laboratory amplifier and recording galvanometer. The square wave signal is a small constant voltage switched on and off. Through manipulation of electronic filters, the low frequency response (top panels) and the high frequency response (lower panels) of the amplifier may be limited at the frequencies indicated (A through I). Limiting of low frequency response causes the top of the square wave to sag, showing that the system is not maintaining response to a steady-state input signal. Contraction of the high frequency range, on the other hand, slows the rise rate of the leading edge of the step function and rounds the corners of the square wave. Slight overshoot at the top corners, probably due to momentum of the recording pen, is present when high frequency response is extended to 75 Hz. Note that decrease of high frequency response abolishes overshoot. Grass 7C system; curvilinear chart paper at 10 mm/sec. Recorded September 30, 1977, with the kind assistance of John Savarese, M.D.

---

*Damping is defined later in this chapter. See also Performance Testing, Chapter 5.

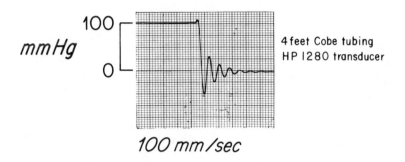

100 mmHg **0**

4 feet Cobe tubing
HP 1280 transducer

100 mm/sec

Figure 1-2 Transient Response of Catheter-Manometer System   Ringing is observed in transient test of grossly underdamped pressure recording system. (See Chapter 5 for methodology.) Resonant frequency of this system is about 27 Hz, with damping factor (beta) of about 0.16.

Harmonic analysis may be applied to nonsinusoidal waves and pulses. It is said that a fundamental frequency plus the first five harmonics will generate a reasonably accurate facsimile of any pulsatile physiologic phenomenon, and that even a square wave can be synthesized from a limited number of frequencies. What the physiologist may consider an acceptable synthetic square wave, however, is grossly distorted by standards applied to music-reproducing equipment of only mediocre quality.

Though perhaps more pertinent to music than to physiology, it is observed that perception of waves and wave phenomena depends on qualities somewhat more subjective than the physical criteria noted so far. A pure sine-wave electronic signal converted into sound is colorless and monotonous. Electronic organs, pianos, and carillons were not commercially successful until designers considered elements such as attack (the rate of build-up of intensity of the wave envelope), decay, and complex overtones (fractional multiples of the fundamental tone frequency).

Frequency vs Repetition Rate

...The fact that an analysis on the basis of a uniform heart rate is easier to make does not mean that the premise is correct. Much evidence can be quoted for the stand that each pulse is indeed an independent event.

John W. Remington[56]

Physiologists analyzing the frequency spectrum of cardio-vascular phenomena tend to equate heart rate with fundamental frequency. This is dubious reasoning. A struck cymbal produces complex sound waves with frequencies of hundreds and thousands per second. The frequency output is the same whether the cymbal is struck once per second or once every five minutes. Similarly, the frequency components of the systemic pressure pulse are the same, regardless of pulse rate (unless of course, changes in rate effect secondary inotropic and vascular alterations). The frequency spectrum of an event should not be confused with the repetition rate of the event, and bears no fixed relationship to it.

OSCILLATION AND RESONANCE

On a corner near my childhood home was a tall metal post with an enamelled steel street sign at the top. With considerable juvenile effort my friends and I could bend the post just a little. Upon release, the post sprang back past the vertical and continued to sway back and forth for a few seconds. Experiments showed that we could shake this post to-and-fro and make the excursions of the post greater and greater with very little input of energy provided (1) we timed our pushes at precisely the right moment, and (2) each push wasn't too fast or too slow. Though we could make the swings of the post larger and larger (but never succeeded in breaking it off), we found it was very difficult to alter the rate at which the post vibrated.

We didn't know it at the time, but our signpost was an oscillating system. It had a preferred or *natural frequency* of oscillation that was dictated by the combination of (1) springiness or capacitance, and (2) mass or inertance. We had also discovered that the amplitude of oscillation of this system could be greatly augmented by the application of very small inputs of energy provided the energy inputs were at precisely the right frequency and "in phase"* with the motion of the post. The frequency at which the system was most receptive to energy input was the resonant frequency (equal to the natural frequency of oscillation).

If we had thought to measure and make a graph of the displacement of the top of the post as a function of time, the graph would have shown a sine wave. The same would have been true of a graph

---

*Phase will be considered shortly.

of the velocity of the signpost. The two waves would not have coincided, however, because the post's greatest velocity occurred while passing through the perpendicular, while the greatest displacement would be observed at the moment of zero velocity.* Velocity and displacement, therefore, were out of phase.

As we grew up and began driving automobiles some of us had to learn how to free a snowbound car by rocking it back and forth through quick reversals of gears and careful engagement of the clutch. Success called for precise application of power exactly in phase with the car's oscillation. Too little power, or power applied at the wrong time, aborted the car's oscillation; too abrupt application of power resulted in spinning of the wheels. Without necessarily thinking about the phenomenon in precise physical terms, we took advantage of the principle that an oscillating system best responds to increments of energy added in phase with the natural frequency of the system; moreover, the applied force must be matched to the velocity of displacement—a matter of impedance (to be examined shortly).

Man's imagination has long been captivated by the undulations of the sea and its endless echelons of waves crashing on the shore. Miniature models offer analyzable lessons regarding oscillation and resonance in fluid systems. Consider a rectangular cake pan filled halfway to the brim with water: lift one edge of the pan, then drop it. A wave travels across the surface of the water, strikes the opposite edge, and then returns. Undulations continue until the wave action is damped by the friction of the water molecules.

The length of the container and the depth of the water in a rectangular basin determine the natural period of oscillation of the wave. If a wave is already established and one tips the basin at just the right time, the amplitude of the wave can be markedly augmented, again showing that an oscillating system readily accepts energy imparted to it in phase with its natural period of vibration. (It doesn't matter much that the basin is tipped coincident with every second, third, or fourth wave. As long as the energy is imparted in phase with the natural frequency of oscillation, the system readily accepts it.) Rather than the cake pan, consider a gigantic basin 225 feet deep and 160 miles long. Such a basin will have a natural period of oscillation of six hours. The dimensions are those

---

*This relationship defines simple harmonic motion.

of the Bay of Fundy in Nova Scotia. Every twelve hours the lunar tide provides a great shove that is precisely in phase with the to-and-fro volume in the Bay. The result is a range of 50 feet between high and low tide, greater than anywhere else on earth. The tide rise in the open sea or on a flat shore may be only a few feet, but the lunar tidal force acting into the Bay of Fundy results in a gigantic increase in water pressure (a 25-foot elevation relative to mean sea level) owing to the resonance of the system.

A visitor from another planet, attempting to draw conclusions about tidal elevations in the Atlantic Ocean, but limited only to observations in the Bay of Fundy, would indeed derive an erroneous impression. The message here is that the site of observation significantly affects the observed amplitude of perturbation that a given input of energy imposes upon a complex system.

PHASE

Fourteen definitions are listed for "phase" in the unabridged edition of *The Random House Dictionary of the English Language.* Our concern with phase is defined as "a particular stage or point of advancement in a cycle." Put another way, phase refers to a particular point in a cyclic repetitive event characterized by waxing and waning qualities.

If an event is cyclic, then its time dimension is also circular and can be expressed in circular or rotational terms. One complete event requires 360° or 2π radians (one radian being equal to 57.3°).

Phase Relationship and Phase Angle

If two phenomena are occurring at the same repetition rate, but the nadir of one coincides with the zenith of the other, then the events are said to be 180° out of phase. The time relationship between two cyclic phenomena can thus be expressed in terms of "phase angle." In the example of the oscillating signpost, displacement and velocity were 90° out of phase.

When you pump up an automobile tire a considerable volume of air has to be delivered before there is substantial increase in pressure. This is a way of saying that "flow leads pressure" at the input to a capacitive or elastic element. The reverse condition obtains at the input to an inductive or inertial element: in pushing a stalled automobile, the most effort (force) has to be applied when the car's velocity is zero. Once forward motion is established, it requires little force to keep the car moving at a steady velocity. In this case, then, motion lags behind force.

In the examples just cited effort and momentum are causally related, but the maxima and minima of each parameter are temporally out of phase. It is convenient to express the time relationship between the point of maximum amplitude in a pressure (or force) phenomenon and the maximum amplitude of the attendant flow (or velocity) phenomenon as phase angle. In the case of elastic and inertial elements, flow may "lead" pressure by as much as 90° or "lag" pressure by up to 90°.

It is the convention that phase angle is referenced to pressure (or force). Whether the phase angle is positive or negative depends upon whether one must travel forward (positive phase angle) or backward (negative phase angle) in time to reach the analogous flow or velocity stage. In the case of flow into a capacitance (the tire), flow has preceded pressure. From the vantage point of pressure then, one has to travel backwards in time to get to the analogous flow event. Therefore, the phase angle describing this relationship is negative. In the case of flow into an inductance (inertial element), pressure precedes flow; therefore, in moving from the pressure event to the analogous flow event, the phase angle (measuring time) is opening up or rotating in a positive direction.* Thus the phase angle between pressure and flow in a system which primarily exhibits inertance is positive.

Under conditions of steady flow (as with direct current), the relationship between pressure and flow is determined purely by resistance. Capacitance (elastic) and inductance (inertial) effects are nonexistent, and the phase angle is zero. Applying a steady state pressure to a system and observing its flow characteristics, therefore, is a technique for determining the resistive elements in a complex system. On the other hand, "forcing" a system by applying a pulsatile pressure and observing the concomitant flow phenomena

---

*In engineering as in trigonometry, positive angular rotation is counterclockwise, just the opposite of the convention for axis rotation in electrocardiography. In both systems of notation, however, the zero reference for angular rotation is the horizontal "three o'clock" position.

will produce information relating to the capacitance and inertial characteristics of the system.

Negative phase angles characterize most of the physiologic systems that will be dealt with in this text. This suggests that vascular pressure phenomena are conditioned largely by capacitive (as opposed to inertial) elements.

Phase Shift

Phase *angle* describes the temporal relationship between two cyclic phenomena. Phase *shift* signifies there has been a change in that temporal relationship.

When a capacitor is charged and discharged by alternating current the phase angle between voltage and current is minus 90°. If a fluctuating current or any other type of "signal" is processed through more complex networks of inductances and capacitances, changes in phase angle between flow and pressure may occur.

The phasic phenomena of interest may be different modalities such as pressure and flow or voltage and current, or they may be qualitatively similar perturbations but of differing frequency. Complex musical signals, for example, may be altered in their phase relationship during the process of amplification and reproduction because interstage coupling components in the amplifier retard some frequencies more than others. (This indicates that phase shift is a frequency-dependent phenomenon.) The auditory system is sensitive to phase shift, and music will sound distorted if gross phase shift is introduced during amplification.

Phase shift is not always disastrous.* It can be manipulated, neutralized, or at least compensated for by the knowledgeable engineer. In industrial power distribution, for example, the inductances in a large number of motors will introduce phase shift between voltage and current. This shift creates an economically undesirable "power factor" because losses in current distribution

---

*It may not even matter. C.P. Smith, speech processing expert, tells me that phase shift has little effect on the intelligibility of voice as opposed to quality of music.

are out of proportion to the energy utilized.* By adding capacitances to the system (capacitances do not consume energy), the plant engineer can restore the power factor toward unity, effecting more economical utilization of the current supplied to his facility.

Phase shift becomes a problem to reckon with in physiologic measurements when precision timing is of importance. For example, event "m" and event "n" may be sequentially generated out of the same physiologic process such as contraction of the heart.

At their point of origin event "m" may precede "n" by a certain number of milliseconds. Because of qualitative differences in their pulsatile nature and modes of transmission, however, the temporal relationship of "m" to "n" may be significantly altered by the time the events reach the periphery to be captured for observation. Phase shift may have occurred.

The relationship of phase shift to frequency will be explored further in the section on damping. The moral at present is that phase shift in transmission and reproducing systems must be calibrated if there is to be precise timing of the interval between related physiologic events.

IMPEDANCE

All too readily invoked like an incantation, the term "impedance" commonly obfuscates rather than enlightens.

Impedance is a measure of the opposition to change. It is an index of the change in force associated with a change in activity in a system. For example, impedance is the ratio of change in force to change in velocity, or the change in pressure associated with a change in flow. In electricity impedance is the ratio of change in voltage to change in current.

High impedance merely means that a relatively large alteration in effort is required to produce a modest change in activity. High impedance also means that if a slight change in activity, such as flow, *does* occur, it must be associated with a large change in pressure (the force moiety).

---

*Power factor: the cosine of the phase angle between voltage and current.

To say that a hydraulic system has "low impedance" means that it requires very little *change* in pressure to effect significant alterations in flow. Put another way but with more significance relative to the vascular tree: a low impedance system is one that will accept large changes in flow with disproportionately little change in pressure. A high impedance system, on the other hand, is one that manifests great increase in pressure when flow is increased just a bit, or that requires great increases in pressure to bring about small modicums of increased flow. What this means in terms of a pumping system will be explored in Chapter 2.

Impedance comes in two varieties: (1) resistive, and (2) reactive. When the elements opposing change are purely viscous or frictional, then changes in force produce changes in activity that are always directly proportional as well as simultaneous. Such elements are termed "resistances" and their impedances are "resistive." Resistance is constant regardless of changes in flow or pressure.* In contrast, the impedance qualities of capacitive (springy) elements as well as those of inductive (inertial) elements are termed reactive. This is an apt term since such elements "react" to *rate* of change rather than simply offer resistance to change.

The automobile again provides useful analogies. If a motor vehicle is already moving at slow speed on the level, then relatively little effort is required to keep it in motion at the same speed. Only the force necessary to overcome a small constant resistive (frictional) impedance need be applied. To *change* the speed of the car, however, is another matter. Now reactive impedance (inertial in this example) is encountered. The value of reactive impedance is related not only to the mass of the car (a constant) but particularly to the *rate* at which the change of speed is effected. More braking force is obviously required to decelerate a car rapidly than to slow it gradually, while shortening the time to accelerate from a standing start to a given speed requires greater engine effort. Thus the value of reactive impedance is a function of the rate of application of force.

Depending on the arrangement of the various reactive elements of a circuit or system, the impedance to pulsatile or oscillatory flow may be much higher—or much lower—than the opposition to flow afforded by the purely resistive components in that circuit. When

---

*In electricity and ideal fluids.

the system input is largely capacitive, impedance falls with increasing frequency; there may be sharp discrepancy between the opposition to steady-state flow (d.c.) as opposed to pulsatile flow. This behavior is observed in the systemic arterial tree where the resistive component of impedance is about 1,500 units.* Impedance to *pulsatile* flow at the input to the system (at the root of the aorta), however, is only 300 units—and remains remarkably constant despite significant changes in viscous resistance at the periphery of the system.[24]

Reactive impedance, then, is unlike resistive impedance. The latter can be defined by a single number which is the same at all frequencies. The absolute value of a reactive impedance, however, depends on the frequency of the applied force (since frequency is a function of the rate of change of the force). Furthermore, the change produced does not necessarily occur at the same point in time that the force is applied. In other words, cause and effect are not necessarily in phase. The temporal disparity or phase relation between cause and effect is also related to frequency.

Owing to the considerations just stated, definition of a reactive impedance at a specific frequency requires two terms: (1) a specific impedance value in ohms or dyne-cm-sec^{-5}, and (2) a phase angle in radians or degrees. Accordingly, a graph relating the input impedance of a physiologic system to the frequency of excitation is commonly accompanied by a second graph which shows the phase angles at the frequencies of interest.

It follows that impedances cannot be manipulated mathematically by simple arithmetic. Rather, total impedance is the vector sum of resistive and reactive elements in a given system.† It also follows that computations of impedance-related qualities must take into account the phase difference between pressure and flow. This is especially pertinent with respect to computation of power, the product of in-phase pressure and flow, since flow and pressure are commonly *not* in phase when flow is pulsatile. Yanof's comment has great significance relative to clinical measurements discussed later in

---

*The units are dyne-sec-cm^{-5}.

†$Z^2 = R^2 + (X_L - X_C)^2$, where Z = impedance, R = resistive impedance, X_L = inductive or inertial reactance, and X_C = capacitive reactance.

this text: "If a biologist were measuring sinusoidal blood pressure in an animal, using a mercury manometer, and sinusoidal blood flow, using a flow meter which could only measure mean blood flow, then he would not be able to determine the instantaneous impedance or the phase difference between pressure (analogous to voltage) and flow (analogous to current). He would have to use a better instrument."[77] Bluntly stated, it is not correct to apply a term such as "stroke work" to numbers which are derived from measurement systems commonly used clinically; "d.c." work, computed from mean values for flow and pressure, is only part of the story. It is likely that circumstances exist wherein the significant burden on the contracting ventricle is represented by the reactive impedance it "sees" (which we can't measure clinically) rather than by the peripheral *resistive* impedance (which is what mean pressure and flow measures give us).

The types of work performed (pulsatile vs d.c.) are quite different for the two sides of the heart, and much investigation has yet to be carried out to define the power output characteristics of the two ventricles and determine what can be done clinically to optimize performance under varying resistive and reactive loads.

It was pointed out in the paragraphs on phase, that the contributions of reactive and resistive influences in a system can be separated out by noting how the system behaves when subjected to a steady stress, and comparing this response to the behavior of the system when excited by oscillatory energy. The closed-circle breathing circuit in an anesthesia machine is an example of a system designed to have low resistive impedance as well as low reactive impedance. With a spontaneously breathing patient connected to the system the pressure within changes very little despite abrupt variations in flow that range from zero to 60 liters per minute. The hallmarks of low impedance systems are identifiable in this circuit: low viscous resistance achieved through use of large bore tubes and valves with large orifices; reactive impedance minimized by low-intertia valve components in the presence of a large-capacitance rebreathing bag.

The concept of impedance need not be confined to physical systems. Human societies are high impedance systems with respect to new ideas. Intense efforts in terms of political activism, propaganda, advertising money, or military force are required to effect abrupt but relatively modest changes in social conduct. Conversely, sweeping alterations in life style of the populace (such as may occur with natural disasters or economic depression) may be associated with abrupt increases in social pressures that find relief only in riot or revolution.

Impedance Matching

Energy is transferred from system to system most efficiently when the output impedance of the first or driving system precisely matches the input impedance of the second or driven system.

If two systems are in series or follow one another and the output impedance of the first is lower than the input impedance to the second system, then energy will be reflected back into the first system or "source." Energy transfer is inhibited. On the other hand, if the driven stage (second system) input impedance is lower than that of the output impedance of the source (first system), there will be "negative reflections" and energy transfer is again compromised. Only when the output impedance of the driving system matches the input impedance of the driven system will energy transfer from one system to the other be complete.

The best-intentioned of scientists have difficulty in producing a conceptual explanation of "impedance matching" in general and of "negative reflection" in particular. The parable of the Cadillacs and the Volkswagens is offered for illumination of the concept of impedance matching.

The Cadillacs and the Volkswagens. An automobile stopped at an intersection is struck from behind by another car. It is a low-speed collision, so there is no crumpling of metal; moreover, neither driver has a foot on the brake. Therefore, there is no loss of energy by friction. Energy exchange occurs solely through the springiness of the cars' bumpers, modulated by the weight (inertia) of the vehicles. The same type of collision occurs on each of three successive days.

On Day One, the stopped car is a Cadillac sedan. It is struck squarely from behind by a Volkswagen Beetle. What happens? The Beetle merely bounces off the rear of the Cadillac. The latter hardly moves. This is an example of "positive reflection" of energy. The Cadillac, with its great mass and stiff springs, presents a high impedance input, poorly matched to the low impedance output of the light and springy Volkswagen. Energy is thrown back: positive reflection, like a tennis ball bouncing off a brick wall.

On Day Two, a Volkswagen is the stopped car. It is hit from the rear by a Cadillac sedan. The Volkswagen caroms sharply forward into the intersection. As for the Cadillac, it is slowed slightly, but does not give up its forward motion. The Cadillac still retains much of its kinetic energy which has not been transferred to the lighter Volkswagen. Again, an "impedance mismatch" exists, but in this case there is "negative reflection" of energy.

On Day Three, the Volkswagen is struck from behind by another Volkswagen of identical construction and weight. The struck car is propelled forward into the intersection at exactly the same rate of speed formerly possessed by the car hitting it from behind, while the striking car comes to a dead halt. This is perfect matching of impedance with total transfer of power from one system to another.

A similar phenomenon of perfect impedance matching under a variety of conditions is seen in the transfer of energy from mass to mass in the executive toy shown in Figure 1-3.

TAPERED TUBES

What do gramophones, fjords, and Dizzy Gillespie's trumpet have in common? Each is a tapered vessel periodically infested with wave phenomena. Each offers opportunities to examine the complex behavior of waves subjected to constraints that change along the axis of wave propagation.

Amplification in Tapered Tubes

Let us look first at the gramophone. Photographs of recording sessions in the early days of acoustical recording show the musicians clustered in front of the mouth of a giant horn. The horn tapers gradually to a diameter about that of a silver dollar. Tightly stretched across this narrow throat is an elastic diaphragm levered to a metal stylus which in turn is pressed against a revolving plate of wax.

By what mechanism can the pressure of sound waves be so intensified as to produce a replica of their undulations chiseled into a wax disc? The answer lies in the behavior imposed upon a wave of sound pressure as it marches down a tapering tube. The energy

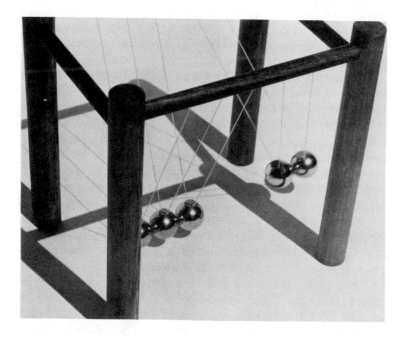

Figure 1-3 Executive Toy (Newtonian Demonstrator) Optimum impedance matching effects complete transfer of energy from driving component to driven component.

content of the wave must remain constant (if frictional losses are discounted). Therefore, as the cross-sectional area of the wave front is progressively constrained, some other factor in the energy equation must increase. Wave velocity in air is also fixed, so the only remaining factor is force per unit area. Force per unit area is pressure—and it is increased. Therefore, a tapered tube will *amplify* the pressure of a wave traveling toward the narrow end. A similar phenomenon is observed in an ocean wave entering a fjord or tapering estuary: the wave gradually increases in height (pressure) as its lateral dimension becomes progressively constrained. Again it is observed that if the energy of the wave is to be preserved when a spatial dimension of the energy envelope is altered, there must follow an equivalent change in the intensity of the wave.

Impedance Matching and Tapered Tubes

Just as the properties of the acoustic horn were utilized to record music, operation of the horn in the reverse direction facilitates re-creation of sound from a mechanical replica embossed in the spiral groove of a phonograph record.

Let us first consider what happens simply if a sewing needle is pressed into the moving groove of a phonograph record. Squeaky, faint sounds may be heard, but the surface of the agitated needle is so small that it simply can't "grab" and disturb much air. As for low tones, these are not reproduced at all. Needle displacement at low frequency is characterized by low velocity, so the needle shaft just slips through the air without creating a ripple, much as a feathered propeller blade or canoe paddle can move through its fluid medium without creating a disturbance.

Next, attach a stiff but lightweight disc or vane to the needle. The vibrating system now has a dimension that is a significant fraction of the wave length of frequencies in the middle of the acoustic spectrum, so more air molecules can be given more of a shove even if the vane moves at low velocity. The sound becomes louder as well as broader in range. Voice reproduced in this manner still sounds tinny, like that of a talking doll (this same mechanism has been used since Edison's day to make toys "talk" or produce sound effects).

A profound improvement in sound quality follows when the phonograph needle is anchored to a diaphragm that occludes the narrow throat of a tapered horn. Now a much broader spectrum of sound is projected from the flaring bell of the horn. High pressure oscillations of air constrained in the narrow throat of the tube have been effectively coupled to a larger volume of air in the room about the listener through the agency of the tapered horn. Finally, using electricity and magnets, a piston capable of high frequency movement can be substituted for the simple mechanical diaphragm. By this mechanism it is now possible to generate very large pressures, indeed, in the throat of the tube; the horn becomes the familiar loudspeaker of public address systems.

Harking back to the concept of impedance, an element characterized by large changes in pressure in the face of lesser changes in displacement can be defined as a high impedance component. On the other hand, large displacements (as a function of time) coupled with modest changes in pressure are the hallmark of low impedance elements. Transferring these definitions to the tapered acoustic horn, the function of the horn is to couple the high impedance diaphragm or piston mechanism at the horn throat to the very low impedance of unconstrained room air at the flaring end of the horn. The horn facilitates the effective translation of energy between components of widely differing impedance. A tapered conduit, then, is an *impedance-matching* element.

Filtering and Resonance in Tapered Tubes

What about the musician's trumpet? Well, horns can do more than reproduce music; they can generate it. Thanks to the constraints inherent in horns, the raucous bray created at the unattached mouthpiece of a brass instrument can be transformed into an amiable musical tone.

Any horn tends to favor certain frequency ranges at the expense of others, owing in part to the resonances of the horn. Such resonances are complex and distributed over a broad range unlike the single resonant frequency of a straight tube such as an organ pipe. The physical dimensions of the horn determine the favored range of frequencies. The sousaphone, a very large horn, translates and embellishes very low frequencies, but the contained column of air simply cannot sustain vibration at middle and high frequencies. In contrast, consider the trombone: shorter and smaller of bore, it manipulates middle frequencies but the very low as well as the very high frequencies are filtered. The air column is not long enough to support extremely low frequency vibrations, nor can its reluctance to vibrate at extremely high frequencies be overcome except through vein-distending effort by the trombonist.

In favoring transmission of a certain range of frequencies while discriminating against frequencies above and below, the horn is a filter. It is a "band-pass" or "broad-band" filter, however, not sharply tuned as in the case of an oscillator that resonates at only a single frequency.*

Characteristic Impedance

Another way of explaining the filtering behavior of horns is to invoke the concept of characteristic impedance. The latter is the

---

*A chime, for example.

impedance of a *specific segment* of a tapered tube. Low at the open bell or flare of the horn, high at the narrow throat at the other extremity, the impedance changes along the length of the horn.

The general rule is that wherever an impedance discontinuity exists, energy reflections occur. The impedance changes in a tapered tube are gradual, so strong reflections are not obvious. Yet, reflections do occur, and reflections mean compromise of power transfer. Since impedance is frequency-dependent, it follows that frequencies above and below certain broad bounds may not be well-accepted by a particular horn. Expressed another way, the energy input to the system at the mouthpiece will not be transferred owing to impedance mismatch. To cite extreme examples, the tight lip of the cornetist is a very high impedance source. The energy of this musician's high notes, if injected into the much lower impedance of the giant sousaphone, will simply dissipate as negative reflections. Conversely, the sousaphonist applying his slack-lipped embouchure to the trumpet will find that the small, high impedance horn throws back his mismatched effort in the form of inelegant noise at the mouthpiece

In summary, tapered conduits possess several properties that affect energy passed through them. First, waves will be amplified in passing from the large to the small end of a tapered conduit. Second, a tapered tube may provide impedance-matching, serving as an effective coupling mechanism between elements having markedly different dynamic properties. Third, the tapered tube is a relatively broad band filter.

DAMPING

An oscillating system does not consume energy. A perfect oscillator, once set in motion, would continue to vibrate throughout eternity. In the real world no perfect oscillator exists. Friction is everywhere: in the sliding of the metal crystals in a spring; between the water molecules in an ocean wave; and in the air resistance offered a swinging pendulum. Any oscillating system, therefore, grinds more or less slowly to a halt as energy is lost in the form of heat created by friction. Damping is a measure of the tendency to stop oscillating.

While damping is related to both the inertance and stiffness of the system, it is essentially a measure of the frictional force acting in opposition to movement of the mass of the system.[22] Inasmuch as capacitance and inertance can affect damping, it follows that damping is another frequency-related parameter.

Damping comes in three grades: critical, optimum, and underdamping.* A *critically-damped* system has a damping factor of one and does not resonate at all. When struck, agitated, or otherwise bent out of position and then released, the movable element returns fairly quickly to equilibrium with no overshoot. When excited by sinusoidal signals such a system has a frequency response curve† that begins to droop early as the input signal frequency is swept from low to high (Figure 1-4). The relative amplitude response has declined by 50% at what would be the undamped resonant frequency of the system. A well-sprung, heavy automobile with good shock absorbers might be an acceptable example of a critically-damped system.

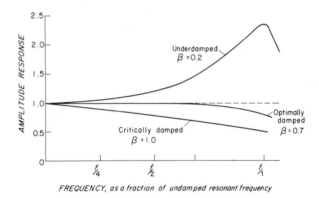

Figure 1-4   Frequency response curves associated with various degrees of damping/β = damping factor.

In contrast, the grossly *underdamped* system has a damping factor that approaches zero rather than one. Once set in motion an underdamped system will continue to vibrate at its resonant frequency for a considerable period of time. A Chinese gong and a car with bad shock absorbers are appropriate analogies.

---

*Strictly speaking, damping is a continuum, but these are qualitative regions of interest.

†A frequency response curve is a graph of the amplitude of the system output vs frequency when the system is excited by a signal of constant intensity but ever-increasing frequency.

Frequency response characteristics of underdamped systems are unlike those of the critically-damped system. If the damping factor is only 0.2 and the system is excited by a sinusoidal signal, the response is "flat" (faithful within 5%) only up to a frequency which is 20% of the undamped resonant frequency. As the test frequency increases, amplitude response increases abruptly, peaks at the resonant frequency, and then sharply drops off so that there is virtually no response to still higher input frequencies. The peakiness at resonance means that the system will demonstrate marked amplitude overshoot (as much as 150%) when excited at its resonant frequency.

As for the *optimally-damped* system, this is one that, when stressed and released, rapidly reverts to its resting position, overshoots very slightly, returns in the other direction, and then comes to rest. Such a system will have a frequency response curve which is flat (within 2% in this case) up to 67% of the undamped natural frequency. Near the undamped resonant frequency, moreover, the amplitude response does not peak, but simply declines rather sharply.*

Manipulation of damping can radically alter the performance of a resonant system in two somewhat related ways. First, an increase in damping degrades high frequency response, just as the drummer's fingers on the edge of a struck cymbal take the sizzle out of the tone. Second, an increase in damping may sharply lower the resonant frequency of the system if the damping change is due to a reduction in stiffness of the system, i.e., the system compliance or capacitance is increased. The result again is loss of high frequency response.

Through manipulation of damping a system may be made to look or sound better than it really is. In the old days, for example, when automobiles had frames and the bodies were made of sturdy metal, a car door would slam shut with a solid thunk. Later, when manufacturers took away the frames and began rolling the sheet metal thinner and thinner, the slamming door sounded "tinny" and much of the car rattled. This destroyed the image of a supposed quality product, so builders lined the doors, the hood, and other

---

*Strandness & Sumner, citing McDonald, regard 0.707 as optimum damping, while I.T. Gabe considers a damping factor of 0.64 as optimal.[68] [20]

expanses of sheet metal with blankets of vibration-damping material. Damping, therefore, may give the superficial appearance of improving an otherwise tinny or peaky system. This is accomplished, however, at the expense of the high frequency response of the system and is often a dodge for covering up the inadequacies of a system of inherently poor quality. The investigator working with a system that "rolls off" in the middle frequencies (owing to damping) may never even be aware of the presence of high frequencies in the experimental preparation.

The approved method of avoiding overshoot, peaking, or ringing in a recording system is to be certain that the resonances of the system are far out into the high frequency region, far beyond those of any frequency of interest. Unhappily this may not be feasible in the clinical setting. As discussed in Chapter 3, the fault lies not so much with the recording devices but with the hydraulic connecting systems.

While an undamped system may ring, phase shift is minimal. Damping introduces phase shift. This is of no importance in the clinical observation of blood pressure amplitude but could significantly affect estimations of time intervals. In an optimally damped system, phase shift is linearly related to frequency, so that correction for phase shift (time delays) is relatively simple.

In summary, damping affects the frequency-response characteristics of a resonant system. Damping is influenced by inertance and by capacitance, the same factors that control resonant frequency. Damping, however, is markedly influenced also by viscosity (friction), a factor that does not appear in the formula for computation of the undamped resonant frequency of a hydraulic system.

The actual formulas are (from Gabe):[20]

(4) For damping factor, beta:

$$\beta = \frac{4\mu}{r^3} \sqrt{\frac{1}{\pi E}}$$

(5) For resonant (natural) frequency, f_0:

$$f_0 = \frac{1}{2\pi} \sqrt{\frac{\pi r^2 E}{\varrho l}}$$

Where

ϱ = density of liquid
l = length of catheter or tubing
r = radius of catheter or tubing
μ = liquid viscosity
E = stiffness of the system, i.e.,
$\frac{\text{change in pressure}}{\text{change in volume}}$;
Note that E is the reciprocal of compliance or capacitance which is: charge or volume/pressure.

For comparison, the resonant frequency of an electrical circuit (f) is given by:

(6)

$$f = \frac{1}{2\pi\sqrt{L \cdot C}}$$

Where

L = inductance
C = capacitance

Filters

Allusion has been made to filtering as a property of horns and other physical systems. There will be considerable discussion of the filtering effects of electronic as well as hydraulic systems later in this text. Some basics about filters are thus in order.

In medicine and in chemistry we tend to think of filters in terms of pore size, like sieves: the smaller the pore, the more selective the filter. Such thinking may be appropriate with respect to particulate substances in a fluid vehicle, but electronic filters need not operate that way; the hierarchical concept is not the only option. Electronic filters can be specific and selective in their activities by design or inadvertence. The tone controls on sound systems are familiar examples of the versatility of electronic filters requiring but a few cents' worth of components.

Filters may be "high-pass" meaning that low frequencies are selectively attenuated, or "low-pass" to indicate attenuation of frequencies above a certain point in the spectrum. A "narrow band" filter attenuates all *except* a short segment of the frequency spectrum. A "notch filter" on the other hand cuts out a narrow locus of frequencies.

A filter is described with respect to (a) where it operates in the frequency spectrum, and (b) the slope of attenuation or roll-off wrought on the signal. The operating point is the frequency at which the signal is attenuated by 50% (or is 3 db down) relative to the flat portion of the frequency response curve.* As for rate of attenuation, a typical low pass music filter might have a roll-off of 6 db per octave, meaning that with each doubling of frequency the signal is reduced to one-fourth of its previous intensity. This is a relatively gentle slope. Selective filters have slopes as steep as 60 db per octave.

MAGIC WORDS

"When *I* use a word," Humpty Dumpty said, in rather a scornful tone, "it means just what I choose it to mean—neither more nor less."

"The question is," said Alice, "whether you *can* make words mean so many different things."

"The question is," said Humpty Dumpty, "which is to be master—that's all."

Lewis Carroll: *Through the Looking Glass*

Contractility

Contractility is not happily or easily defined. The word "does not have a very precise meaning," note Leonard and Hajdu.[42] Definitions "abound," they say, so the word "contractility" has

---

*The db or decibel scale is a logarithmic index of intensity employed in acoustics and in signal processing. Intensity discrimination capability is not acute inasmuch as biologic sensors tend to operate logarithmically, and a 50% reduction in intensity is required before the listener can detect a change.

28

"various meanings for various investigators. Isometric tension, iso-
tonic shortening, velocity of shortening, cardiac output, stroke work,
efficiency, all have been measured in the name of contractility..."

Leonard and Hajdu define contractility in terms of a length-
tension or work diagram; there is no consideration of velocity or
power.[42] That is, contractility is a measure of work (force times
distance), whether the work is accomplished rapidly or slowly.

Albeit authoritative, the strict construction employed by
Leonard and Hajdu seems inadequate as a clinical concept of contractility owing to the absence of a time consideration.[42] Almost invariably work costs more when it is done quickly than if accomplished slowly, whether one is building a house, buying electricity, or
pumping blood. Our clinical concerns in applying monitoring
techniques in the care of the severely ill lie with the cost of cardiac
work. That cost seems to be related to the *style* in which the ventricle
performs a given aliquot of work. (This seems more and more evident in the evolving use of vasodilator therapy and drugs such as
propranolol.) Clinically at least, a definition of contractility should
embrace the concept of performance, as opposed simply to a quan-
tum of work accomplished without consideration of time.*

I find it more satisfactory, therefore, to define contractility in
terms of a family of curves relating tension to velocity of fiber
shortening. Enhanced contractility means that the isolated muscle
can lift a given weight more rapidly, or that it requires no increase in
time to lift a greater weight the same distance.†

I will use inotropism as almost synonymous with contractility
except that inotropism will refer more to ostensible behavior and

---

*Work is the product of volume and pressure. Power, an index of perfor-
mance, is work per unit of time, or the product of pressure and flow.
†One of the best statements of the factors affecting apparent cardiac performance is presented by Sonnenblick and Strobeck (except that their definition of power is wrong).[64] Contractility is defined as a "surface" [three-
dimensional graph] "generated during contraction by the interrelated
variables of force, velocity, and length at any instant..."See also Braunwald.[7] "The *limits* to mechanical performance" (say Sonnenblick and
Strobeck), "whether force development or shortening, are set by the level of
contractility, but what the muscle actually does within these limits depends
on the initial loading (pre-load) that sets the muscle-fiber length and instantaneous loading during the contraction (afterload)."

performance, while contractility applies largely to the intrinsic capabilities of ventricular muscle. Strictly speaking, contractility is a quality, while inotropism is an influence or modifier (*ino-* = fiber, *-tropos* = a turning, influencing; ergo: inotropic = influencing the contractility of muscular tissue). The terms have come to be used virtually interchangeably, a semantic error that I am deliberately guilty of perpetuating in this text.

Afterload

Afterload has been considered clinically equivalent to vascular resistance, intramyocardial systolic tension, ventricular wall tension, and aortic impedance. Afterload can't be all these at the same time. It is, in fact, none of the above.

Afterload is defined in terms of a laboratory preparation: the weight which an isolated papillary muscle is obliged to lift upon electrical stimulation while velocity of contraction is recorded. (The weight is constant throughout a given contraction.) Caution must be exercised in transferring this concept to the intact vascular system.

If it must be adapted as a clinical concept, afterload may be tenuously analogous to ventricular wall tension. Tenuously, because laboratory afterload is a constant during contraction while ventricular contraction involves time-dependent variables: (1) wall tension at a given intracavitary pressure decreases as the radius of the cavity becomes smaller, and (2) the pressure in the ventricle increases during contraction. Furthermore, *rate* of change of pressure is not related to peripheral resistance. The rate of change of pressure is determined by (a) the rate of change of volume, and (b) the input impedance to the aorta.

Not only is afterload in that category of magic words such as patriotism and grounding—impressive facades with elastic meanings—but its use also fosters ambiguity, particularly since electrical models and analogies are commonly promoted for analysis and understanding of cardiovascular phenomena. The intended meaning of afterload is in fact exactly the opposite of the concept of load in electricity. A heavy electrical load is one that has *low* resistive impedance and draws greater current from the source, lowering supply voltage (pressure). The ultimate heavy load is a short circuit. Conversely, a light load in the electrical sense has *high* resistance, draws little current (flow), and maintains a higher voltage at the source.

The ultimate light electrical load is an open circuit with infinite peripheral resistance. (Contrast this with high peripheral systemic vascular resistance which is considered a *large* afterload.)

SUMMARY

Oscillation is commonly encountered in both natural and mechanical systems owing to the concomitant presence of mass (inertia) and springiness (compliance). Each system comprised of these components will have a characteristic frequency at which it prefers to vibrate. This is the resonant frequency and is determined by the product of inertia and compliance.

An oscillating system will vibrate with increased vigor if small increments of energy are added to it in phase and at a frequency that precisely matches the resonant frequency.

Damping is a measure of the tendency of an oscillating system to come to rest owing to loss of energy through friction. An underdamped system tends to "ring" at its resonant frequency when excited by an external force. An increase in damping can have the effect of markedly lowering the frequency response of a resonant system.

Pressure amplification of wave disturbances is seen in natural and mechanical systems. The undulations of waves of low pressure but broad front, such as hydraulic or sound waves, can be converted into waves of higher pressure if confined to narrowing channels.

Phase shift occurs in passing through transmission or amplification systems. This means that the time relationship between waves of differing frequencies will be altered.

Impedance is a measure of resistance to change and is of significance with respect to the optimum transfer of energy between systems and components of systems. Energy that is not transferred owing to an impedance mismatch is reflected.

Semantic imprecision leads to difficulties in communication, diversion of comprehension, and problems with interpretation of experimental observations. Words and concepts utilized in the remainder of the text have been defined in this chapter.

How to evaluate and calibrate the characteristics of oscillating systems will be discussed in Chapter 5 in the section on testing of systems used for direct measurement of pressure.

2 Considerations in the Design of a Pumping System

Ezekiel saw a wheel,
Way up in the middle of the air.
Ezekiel saw a wheel,
Turnin',
Way in the middle of the air.

And the big wheel run by faith,
And the little wheel run by the grace of God.
Was a wheel in a wheel,
Way in the middle of the air.

> Spiritual inspired by the vision of the Prophet Ezekiel.

The evolutionary trend of life has been toward greater mobility and agility. The development of vascular systems and high blood flow has been essential to this evolutionary trend...

> A.J. Marengo-Rowe

For blood to flow, there must be a pump. The most useful of pumps is the turbine. Valveless, with but one moving part, the turbine will provide flow adjustable over a wide range. Save for the report in the first chapter of Ezekiel, and possibly in the ciliary motors of bacteria, rotatory motion on a bearing has not been observed in nature.[6] To meet evolutionary demands then, what alternative might be contrived as a pump for the circulatory system of a mobile beast? After countless trials, a pump design suitable for both man and mastodon evolved: a folded tube, chambered and valved, encased in a chunk of modified striated muscle.

Though warranted for more than the violent lifetimes of its earlier owners, a muscular pump presents several functional problems. The discharge of energy in striated muscle occurs in short pulses, with a disproportionately long reset time between each

31

pulse. Moreover, muscle contraction is an all-or-none phenomenon, and muscle fibers generally react poorly to challenges that force a slower rate of contraction. The intermittent quality of muscle action is also dictated by the consideration that a contracted muscle tends to shut off its own blood supply. (Note how the competitive lifter of weights literally jerks the heavy barbell from the floor, pausing with the weight at chest level; then another intense effort hoists the weight overhead.)

Additional severe handicaps accrue if a pulsatile pump is obliged to discharge directly into a complex of narrow tubes offering a viscous resistance. First, the mass of fluid in the system comes to a halt at the end of each pulse, and the entire liquid contents of the system require reacceleration with the next pump stoke. Second, unmoderated and impulsive discharge of energy is accompanied by great swings of pressure in the pump and in the discharge vessels—pressure swings that are far above and below whatever mean pressure is required to achieve satisfactory flow through the peripheral resistance elements. Such a pump must do a great deal of work simply generating pressure while moving little volume. Net power output will be low. This type of work (pressure work) is peculiarly costly in terms of fuel and oxygen consumed by muscle.*

It does not make good engineering sense, then, to have a strongly pulsatile energy source working into a fixed resistive element. At one extreme of effort, the pump may simply stall; emptying is so compromised that the pump can't refill for the next stroke. At the other extreme, when the power source is still strong enough to produce very high bursts of energy despite intense back pressure, some of the energy will go into setting up spurious vibration, just as an automobile engine will knock or ping under stress. Moreover, the purpose of the heart is merely to generate flow for the transport of fuel and oxygen to the periphery. The body does not run on power generated by the heart. The function of the heart is unlike a dynamo which actually generates a commodity (power) that is conveyed to peripheral sites of consumption. The only power demand on the heart arises from the purely incidental consideration that peripheral

---

*Work is the product of pressure and volume. Power is the rate of doing work and is equal to the product of in-phase pressure and flow.

distribution channels are required to be of small bore and have modest internal pressure owing to local considerations having to do with effective diffusion.

For a muscular heart to operate for even a brief period, some mechanism must be provided for converting pulsatile flow into more or less continuous flow. For the system to operate with any degree of longevity, the flow conversion must be rendered efficient; that is, it should require the least consumption of power by the heart. Since power is the product of flow multiplied by pressure, but the flow moiety (cardiac output) is fixed by metabolic needs, then the key to optimizing cardiac efficiency lies in measures to minimize wide pressure swings around whatever average pressure is required to sustain adequate peripheral flow.

Toward developing an appreciation for the ingenious physiologic solution to this complex engineering challenge, it is worthwhile to reflect that the history of man's development of machines is interlaced with a similar problem: that of translating intermittent motion into continuous motion. Mechanical models displayed in museums of science and industry give a sense of the number of options available and the cleverness exercised. Flywheels, springs, and dashpots were the initial ways of slowing down and smoothing out the discharge of energy from sources of intermittent power. In the age of the internal combustion engine and of rockets, antiknock compounds and slow-burning fuels allow machines to run more efficiently by controlling the explosion within the combustion chamber.

But slowing down the discharge of energy is a dodge not available to cardiac muscle.* What kind of hydraulic mechanism *can* be contrived to convert the pulsatile energy of muscular contraction into continuous flow? Again turning to man's machines, we find that an effective mechanism was developed during the

---

*Increasing the force opposing mechanical systole does, indeed, significantly slow the rate of fiber shortening, while sympathetic stimulation increases velocity of contraction.[7] Practically speaking, however, the duration of mechanical systole is always brief (about 300 milliseconds), and is but a small fraction of the time that blood flow is continually utilizable by the tissues. Moreover, two-thirds of the volume ejected from the ventricle is displaced in the first 100 milliseconds of systole.[75]

Industrial Revolution. The contrivance is seen in its most elegant form in the fire pumps that came into widespread use in the 1800s. Fiercely competitive fire brigades rushed hand tubs to 19th century conflagrations. Many of these fine machines are still in existence (Figures 2-1 through 2-6) and are exercised in a more friendly spirit of competition at firemen's musters. Observing these exercises provides lessons on the best way—developed through much trial and error—of coupling intermittent muscular activity to a hydraulic system delivering continuous flow.

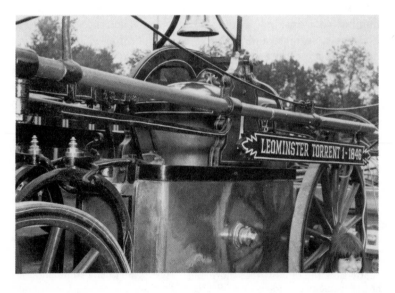

Figure 2-1 Hand tub   A cast brass tub is a prominent feature of this elegantly restored specimen. The wooden spar, one of two hand grips, is folded in its traveling position against the side of the machine. A heavy rocker arm arcs over the air chamber.

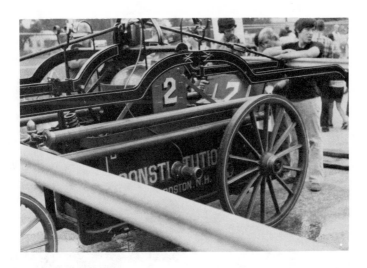

Figure 2-2   Hand tub "Constitution" from New Boston, New Hampshire
Boy is leaning on one of two spars that provide hand grips for the pump
team. As many as 60 men operate these machines to generate pressures of
200 lb/in^2 (10,000 torr) and project a stream of water 200 feet.

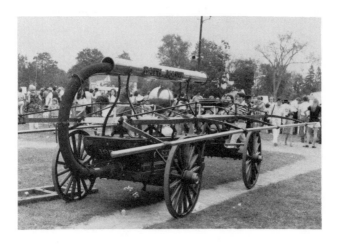

Figure 2-3   Hand tub   Large pipe, sweeping overhead in stowed position,
draws water from cistern or pond.

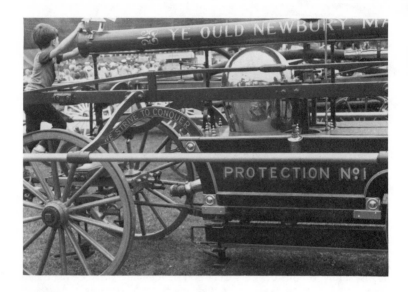

Figure 2-4 Hand tub Then as now, the fierce pride the proprietors of the hand tubs attached to their work and machines is reflected in elegant craftsmanship, exhortive slogans, august titles, and immaculate maintenance.

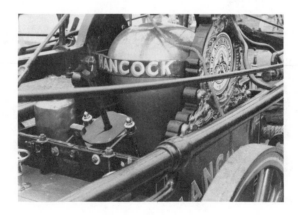

Figure 2-5 Hand tub "Hancock" of Ashburnham, Massachusetts Air chamber is prominent feature. Foregound: one of two pump cylinders. The other is at opposite end of tub. The two operate reciprocally, linked through massive rocker arm that arches over chamber.

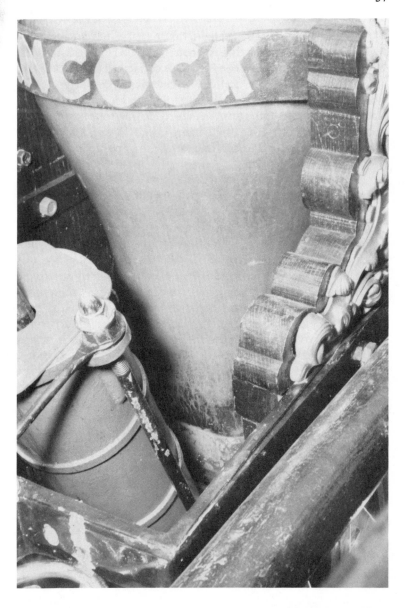

Figure 2-6 Hand tub "Hancock" Pump cylinder discharges through check valve, almost directly into air chamber astride outflow pipe to hose coupling.

The fire pumps are called hand tubs because they are manually operated and the main body is shaped like a tub (Figure 2-1).* The pump has two cylinders. The pistons are connected to a rocker arm so that they operate reciprocally. Wooden spars connected to extensions of the rocker arm provide handholds for groups of men positioned on each side of the tub. The hearty downstroke of one group causes compression in one of the pump cylinders, sucks water from the tub into the other cylinder, and raises the opposite handbar to a position of readiness for a downstroke by the cohorts on the opposite side.

A large metal chamber, shaped rather like a pear standing on its narrow end, sits astride a short outlet pipe that joins the two cylinders to the hose connection (Figure 2-5). The chamber is largely filled with air. As water is ejected from one pump cylinder via a check valve, a little goes toward the fire hose connection. Most of the volume of ejected water, however, takes the easier route into the air chamber. The rapidly rising water level progressively compresses the air above it. When the piston downstroke is completed and the check valve closes, the compressed air in the chamber drives the stored water volume back out of the chamber into the fire hose and out of the hose nozzle.

The compression chamber markedly affects the operation of the man-powered pump with respect to (a) demand for energy, and (b) character of fluid output. It does this by allowing the pumping system to accept abrupt inputs of volume with disproportionately little change in pressure. Expressed another way, the compression chamber permits the pressure head in the system to undulate modestly about a mean despite the fact that pressure and flow in the pump cylinders change precipitously in the course of each muscle-powered stroke.

These considerations render the hand tub a useful fire-fighting implement when power must be supplied by muscular effort. Owing to the compression chamber, the fireman at the hose nozzle is furnished a fairly steady stream of water that may be targeted more accurately onto the blaze. As for the men who supply the muscle

---

*Later versions shown in Figures 2-3 and 2-4 were provided with large intake hoses to draw water from cisterns, ponds, or water mains.

power, the advantages that accrue to them are several. For one thing it is not necessary to restart the water volume in the entire hose system with each stroke. The only water mass to be accelerated is that contained in the pump cylinder. Fluid is always flowing out of the discharge hose as the compression chamber utilizes energy stored in the overlying air during the preceding pump stroke. The compression chamber also gives the pump men a purely mechanical boost. This comes about because there is slightly less back pressure in the system at the initiation of the downstroke when the men have their arms over their heads and are at a mechanical disadvantage. Later in the stroke as the chamber pressure approaches its peak, the bar approaches its lowest point and the men can literally put their bodies into the effort (see Figure 2-7). The best mechanical advantage is thus achieved at the moment of encountering greatest opposition (afterload?).

Of paramount importance is the fact that the compression chamber substantially enhances the efficiency of muscle as an energy conversion mechanism.* The chamber does this by allowing the pump men to accomplish all the work of a given stroke without constraint of time against an opposing force that increases relatively little during a given stroke. In other words the effect of the compression chamber is to maximize displacement of volume while minimizing the time that tension must be sustained.

In order to appreciate better the significance of the previous statement, let's digress a moment and look at the concepts of (a) mechanical work, and (b) muscle as an energy conversion system. Mechanical work is simply the product of force (tension) multiplied by distance (displacement). Merely sustaining tension accomplishes no work in the external mechanical sense. On the other hand, muscle is obliged to consume fuel and oxygen in just maintaining tension. This means that energy is converted to heat even though shortening is prohibited and no useful mechanical work is performed.

In bookkeeping terms there are two line items in the debit column of the energy conversion budget for muscle. The first item is the energy cost of sustaining tension. That cost is directly

---

*Efficiency of a mechanical or electrical system is the ratio of power output to power input. (Power is work per unit of time.)

40

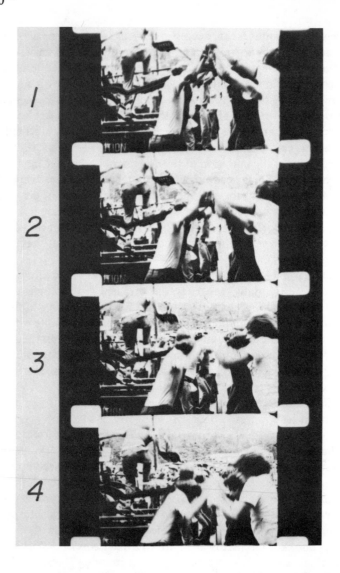

Figure 2-7 Motion Picture Sequence: Firemen's Muster Team Pumps Hand tub at Maximum Effort Owing to the very low reactive impedance offered by the capacitance vessel, little change in pressure accompanies the drastic changes in ejection velocity that occur in the course of each stroke. Put another way, the marked change in flow that occurs between frames 1 and 5 does not mandate a great increase in muscle tension.

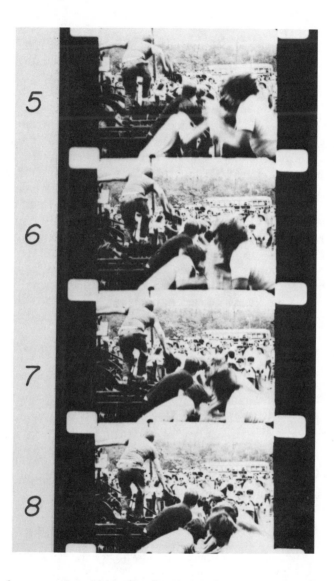

Peak pressure is reached after flow is largely complete. Note optimum mechanical advantage at this point (frames 6 and 7 vs frame 1).

Photographed at 16 frames per second. Shutter speed of 1/30 second blurs rapid motion in middle frames. Team captain, top left in each frame, rides rocker arm that links pictured group with reciprocating cohorts. It is purely coincidence that this tube is stroked at one cycle per second, exactly eight frames encompassing one downstroke.

proportional to time and to tension. The second line item is the cost of shortening (against tension which has already been paid for, so to speak, by the first item). In looking for ways of effecting economy in energy conversion, there is not much that can be done by altering shortening inasmuch as this is a determinant of work. As for the cost of tension, though, that increases almost directly with time. Yet time is not a determinant of work. Therefore, reducing the time factor in the product of tension and time will not compromise work but will directly effect economy in the energy conversion budget.

The message from the previous paragraphs: if work has to be performed requiring a certain tension in order to effect a particular amount of displacement, it makes physiologic sense (in terms of efficiency of energy conversion) to accomplish the work as quickly as practicable.

Some examples may offer reassurance that this is not a something-for-nothing con game. When you hold your arms outstretched motionless for ten full minutes, you technically perform no work. But how do your muscles feel? Have you paid a price in terms of energy utilization?

Another example: if you have to help move a heavy patient, the force you must exert is a constant established by gravity acting on the mass of the patient. It is not in your best interest to spend ten seconds slowly elevating the patient when you can do the same work with less sweat in three seconds. (But gently, please!)

Analogies and arguments have been offered in support of the following premise.

Efficiency dictates that the tension-time product* of a muscle-driven pump be minimized. It is possible to do this without compromising work because work is determined solely by the produce of displacement and pressure.

---

*The tension-time product is similar to tension-time index which is the area under a curve depicting ventricular pressure as a function of time. The tension-time product is not to be confused with max dp/dt, a measure of the contractile state of muscle. An increase in the latter index is associated with increase in fuel expenditure and oxygen demand for the same amount of work.[63] Dp/dt is a matter of the style of muscular contraction which will be examined in Chapter 3. The present discussion deals with muscle of given contractile capability subjected to externally imposed performance constraints.

Minimizing the tension-time product is the function of the compression chamber on the hand tub. The chamber relieves the pump men of any constraint of time on a given stroke. The compression chamber accomplishes this by permitting the system to accommodate large changes in volume with relatively little change in pressure. Put another way, the compression chamber allows the pump cylinder's ejection velocity to be adjusted to the contractile mechanism of muscle without paying a large price in terms of increased pressure. This facilitates maximum conversion of energy into displacement of volume rather than the mere sustaining of tension.

The energy savings brought about by a pump design that increases muscular efficiency are substantial. The magnitude may be appreciated by applying numbers to a typical fire pump. Assume that, at a working pressure of 200 lb/in^2, the hose nozzle discharges in one second a fluid volume equal to the displacement of one pump cylinder. (This means that the hand tub must be stroked once per second.) If there were no compression chamber and the cylinder discharged directly against the resistance of the hose and nozzle, then the pump men depressing the bar would be required to produce immediately at the onset of each stroke a pressure of 200 lb/in^2; then, depressing the bar at constant velocity throughout the stroke, they would be obligated to sustain exactly the same pressure for one full second. On the other hand, pumping at the same rate but with a compression chamber in the system, velocity of displacement could be adjusted over a wide range with little resulting change in system pressure. Freed from restriction on stroke (ejection) velocity, the pump men now are able to complete a downstroke in only half a second.

Let's look at what this means in terms of energy cost. The stroke work of the pump is the same when a given volume is displaced from the hose nozzle at a stipulated pressure whether there is a compression chamber or not, but the amount of obligatory energy conversion by muscle to produce the same external work is quite different in the two types of pump. While peak pressure may have to be increased by about 15% in order to maintain a stipulated mean pressure if there is a compression chamber, the chamber allows reduction of the *time* that muscle must be under tension during a given stroke. By cutting the tension-time product (index) nearly in half, the compression chamber allows a 50% reduction in that portion of the energy budget appropriated to sustaining muscle tension.

For the same stroke work, efficiency of energy conversion is markedly enhanced.

In summary, a price is paid in terms of energy conversion by muscle when tension is generated whether or not displacement is accomplished. Efficiency dictates that duration of tension be minimized in favor of displacement. This end is served when a muscular generator of pulsatile flow is permitted to eject its stroke volume into a vessel that accommodates large changes in flow with little change in pressure.

The compression chamber of the antique hand tub is, of course, a capacitance. Serving the function termed impedance-matching, the capacitance presides over the efficient transfer of power.* In general physical terms, transfer is from the power source—the muscle-driven piston at one end of the system—to the power sink at the other end where power is dissipated in flow through resistance. The smoothing function or filtering action of the capacitance tends to be obvious, but it should not eclipse the importance of the capacitance in transferring power and rendering the system more efficient.

Impedance is a measure of how difficult it is to change things (Chapter 1). It is the ratio of change in pressure to change in flow. The muscle-powered piston pump represents a low impedance energy source characterized by large orifices and minimal friction. Relatively little change in pressure is required to effect relatively large changes in flow through the pump cylinders. The hose and nozzle, on the other hand, represent a high impedance that is wholly frictional (resistive) in character. Through this resistance every increase in flow requires a proportional increase in pressure.

It is one of the axioms of engineering that energy transfer is compromised when the output impedance of the driving system is different from the impedance at the input to the driven system. In the case of the fire pump, the large capacitance chamber immediately downstream from the pump cylinder permits the cylinder to "look into" or "see" an impedance that is relatively low at the cycling rate involved. (Impedance is a frequency-dependent function.)

---

*I deliberately shift terminology at this point from work to power, because power is the more appropriate measure of performance. Work and stroke work say nothing about rate of energy conversion.

On the other hand, looking back upstream from the viewpoint of the hose and nozzle, the source appears to be the pressure chamber which now somewhat resembles a high impedance element in that a modest increase in flow (as might be effected by changing to a larger nozzle) would result in marked drop in pressure.

While the impedance match is not perfect, power transfer is far more effective than it would be without the capacitance. I have already remarked on the cost of *sustained* effort that would be required of the pump men if the stenosis represented by the hose and nozzle were connected directly to the outflow valve of the pump cylinder for which the men provide muscle power. Thanks to the capacitance chamber, a series of grunts at one end of the system is converted to a gush at the other with optimal efficiency.

Later in the 19th century when steam-powered fire engines came into use, the air chamber was retained. Because it allows marked changes in rate of volume displacement with little resulting change in pressure, the air chamber helps keep the steam piston from stalling against a sudden increase in back pressure and facilitates delivery of a steady stream of water from the hose nozzle. The compression bell or air chamber is seen on the steamer engine in the left foreground of the book jacket print, while in the middle ground a large team of men is stroking a hand tub in cadence with the exhortations of their captain standing astride the tub.

What is the point of so many variations on a theme based on an antique machine? How does a fire engine relate to the circulatory system? The aorta and larger arteries provide a capacitance vessel analogous to the air chamber in the fire pump. Weber in 1834 was so struck by the analogy to the fire pump that he coined the term "windkessel" to describe the dynamic behavior of the arterial pressure pulse.[75] Windkessel literally means "air chamber" and translates as fire engine.*

The existence of a capacitance receptacle for ventricular ejectate elegantly facilitates cardiac efficiency. Consider what would have to happen if the ventricle emptied directly into the peripheral resistance. Peak ventricular outflow normally is upwards of 400 ml/sec. To attain this flow rate into a fixed viscous resistance†

---

*Authoritative translation is owed to Lambertus J. Drop, M.D., Ph.D.
†Of 1,500 dyne-sec-cm^{-5}.

would require that the ventricle develop a pressure of more than 450 mm Hg! Not only would greater ventricular pressure be required for ejection against a purely resistive load, but such a load would also markedly extend the time that tension must be sustained in order to deliver a given stroke volume. Ordinarily, fully two-thirds of the stroke volume is ejected during the first one-third of mechanical systole, and peak ventricular pressure is not reached until ejection flow is largely complete. A fixed resistance to ventricular outflow would distribute flow evenly throughout systole, almost tripling the time that pressure must be sustained in the ventricle.

The lesson: for a given combination of heart rate, output, and mean arterial pressure, the mechanical work accomplished by the heart is the same whether it discharges into a capacitance or into a resistance; but the energy costs are profoundly different. Herein lies the advantage of a capacitant aorta and the lethality of a fixed orifice close to the heart.

Still another consideration bearing on cardiac efficiency relates to the peculiar geometry of ventricular contraction. Unlike a cylinder pump that changes volume solely by change in length of the chamber, the ventricle changes volume largely by change in radius. For a given intracavitary pressure, according to Laplace, "hoop tension" or encircling tension on the wall of a chamber is proportional to the radius of the chamber. Owing to the capacitance of the aorta during mechanical systole, the afterload encountered by the ventricular wall does not peak until cavitary volume is approaching a minimum.* The terminal stroke increase in aortic pressure thus may be achieved with proportionately little further increase in ventricular wall tension.

It turns out that the windkessel circuit (Figure 2-8) is too simple an explanation for all the variations of pulsatile pressure and flow observed in the systemic circulation. Indeed, there is continuing dispute over, and investigation into, just what is an adequate model of the arterial circulation.† Since all the data that would permit writing the definitive program for a computer have not been collected, mathematical modeling has finite limitations as a tool for

---

*Strictly speaking, afterload is a constant load, and the term is misused when applied to the ventricle which sees a continually increasing pressure during systole. See Magic Words, Chapter 1.

†Spencer and Denison's much more satisfactory model is shown in Chapter 3.[65]

understanding the arterial circulation. Still, an appreciation of the windkessel (and the antique hand tub) will bring one a long way toward understanding some of the intricacies of mechanical systole and the resulting perturbations of the vascular tree.

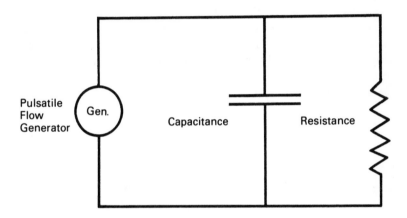

Figure 2-8   Windkessel Circuit

SUMMARY

As a pumping system, the heart and great vessels resemble fire pumps of an earlier era. Windkessel refers to both fire engine and a conceptualization of cardiovascular function.

Muscle converts energy most efficiently when allowed to perform contractile work at a velocity dictated by intrinsic characteristics. When subjected to external constraints on velocity of shortening, as when a muscular pump generates flow against a fixed resistance, fuel and oxygen requirements for work performed are markedly increased.

A low impedance is defined as the facility to accommodate significant flow change with relatively little change in pressure. A low impedance capacitance vessel astride the outflow tract of a pulsatile pump accommodates the stroke ejectate of the pump with little resulting pressure change. This means not only that pressure fluctuations in the discharge system are minimized, but the flow generator is also permitted to optimize its ejection velocity in sympathy with its intrinsic contractile mechanism. Tension-time product is reduced, markedly reducing the energy conversion required of muscle to produce a given amount of stroke work.

Stroke work is not an index of energy conversion by muscle.

In operational terms applied to the arterial tree, impedance to pulsatile flow out of the heart is much smaller than the resistive impedance of the periphery owing to the capacitance provided by the aorta and larger arteries. Large vessels provide impedance matching between a low-impedance flow source and a high-impedance peripheral resistance.

3 The Pressure Pulse

It is generally held that Poisseuille's Law adequately describes the relationship of arterial blood pressure and flow. The basic assumptions underlying his law are that there is steady, laminar, parallel flow of a Newtonian liquid in a straight, smooth-walled tube.

The arterial blood circulation is pulsatile, the fluid is non-Newtonian, and the vessels are of complex geometry and elasticity.

Peterson[54]

What we call the pulse wave is not a wave. A better term is pressure pulse. Its characteristics vary according to where and how it is observed.

Transfer of energy from the ventricle into the aorta is a phenomenon of such complexity that the pressure pulse must be regarded as a composite of several elements even at its genesis. These elements undergo changes in amplitude and time relationship as the pulse moves away from the root of the aorta, traverses the large vessels, and is reflected upon encountering abrupt impedance discontinuities at the periphery. Further modifications occur at the interface with the measuring system and within the measuring system itself. These latter modifiers include the peripheral location of the cannula, the hydraulic connecting system including the transducer, and the amplifier and recording machinery. As it is finally captured for observation on a cathode-ray-tube screen, therefore, the signature of the pressure pulse is quite unlike that at the root of the aorta.

This chapter deals with the creation and the modification of the pressure pulse.

Basic to this discussion is appreciation of the fact that the pressure pulse travels much faster than blood *flows*. The pressure pulse travels 3 to 14 meters per second, about 15 to 100 times the velocity of blood flow.[50] [75] The pressure pulse, therefore, reaches the peripheral arterioles 200 to 300 milliseconds after the onset of ventricular ejection, but the blood ejected during that particular systole does not reach the periphery until several heartbeats later.

At this point it is appropriate to define the ambiguous term systole. This text refers to *pressure* systole unless mechanical systole of the heart is specified. Mechanical systole includes the preejection period of isovolumetric contraction plus the ejection period. There is a significant delay between the initiation of volume ejection and the attainment of systolic pressure in the root of the aorta. The maximum aortic pressure is reached only when flow from the ventricle is largely complete.*

Since pressure systole peaks when mechanical systole is nearly over, pressure is about 60 degrees out of phase relative to flow at the

---

*When listening through an esophageal stethoscope, one hears the "dup" of the second heart sound (signifying end of mechanical systole) at or before the radial arterial pulse tracing reaches its peak. (The observed lag in pressure is, of course, slightly augmented by the transit time for the pressure pulse to reach the periphery.)

aortic root—with flow leading pressure. An out-of-phase relationship is a signal that a capacitance phenomenon is at work, an indicator that we will *not* expect to find a simple linear relationship (as in Ohm's law) between pressure and flow in the vascular system, and a flag of caution regarding ventricular work and power calculations (since power is the product of *in-phase* pressure and flow).

Table 3-1
The Pressure Pulse

	Systolic phenomena		**Manifestation**
Phase One	Early systolic or inotropic phase	:	Probably relate to peak ascending aortic blood flow acceleration	
	Acceleration transient (of Peterson)		Sound wave "Knocking"
	Ejection pulse		Pressure wave
Phase Two	Volume displacement phase		
	Volume displacement component		Fills out and sustains pressure pulse

	Late systolic plus diastolic events	**Manifestations**
Phase Three	Reflection and resonance	Duration of pressure systole
	Discharge of capacitance	Downstroke "Dicrotic notch"
	Runoff	Diastolic waves

COMPONENTS OF THE PRESSURE PULSE

It is convenient to divide the pressure pulse into three phases: (1) early systolic events, (2) midsystolic events, and (3) events of late systole and diastole. These divisions and further subdivisions are shown in Table 3-1 and Figure 3-1. Functionally the divisions correspond to (1) inotropic events, (2) volume displacement, and (3) runoff and reflection. The inotropic events are associated with inscription of the upstroke of the pressure pulse and are probably related to peak ascending aortic blood flow acceleration and to the creation of a true pressure wave. These early events merge with a phase of volume displacement that fills out and sustains the rounded

52

peak of the pressure pulse. Finally, the phenomena of late systole through diastole account for the downturn of the pressure pulse and its further ramp-like decline until the beginning of the next systolic pressure pulse. Runoff, reflections, and true peripheral resistance

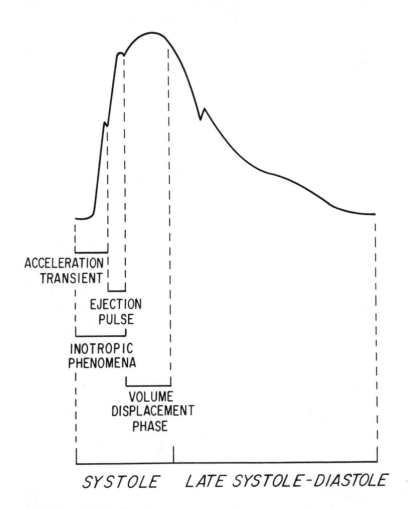

Figure 3-1 Pressure Pulse The time divisions are arbitrary approximations for descriptive purposes. They are not to be confused with the precise event boundaries applied to curves of similar appearance describing, for example, systolic time intervals.

are factors operating here, with various notches and waves imposed upon the systolic down leg and diastolic ramp.

The foregoing three divisions are somewhat arbitrary. Some of the labels for components of the pressure pulse are admittedly novel, but applied with a purpose: in comparing text, illustrations, and tables, it is easier to deal with descriptive labels as opposed to cryptic lettering and numeration systems that must be repeatedly decoded for identification of events under discussion.

Not all the events to be described have been well-characterized. Research in this field has yet to provide answers to many questions. Interpretations offered may in many cases be regarded as tentative.

The Inotropic Component

The purpose of myocardial contraction is to propel blood to the periphery in pulses occurring about once per second. While the pattern of electrical systole organizes and moderates the sequence of contraction, ventricular contraction nonetheless occurs suddenly, almost explosively. So intense is the initial generation of energy by the heart that not all of this energy can be accepted as useful input to the systemic hydraulic system. The situation is akin to an automobile engine that pings when combustion occurs more rapidly than the descending piston can accommodate the expanding gases. The unassimilated energy is reflected back into the engine block as noise and vibration.

The early part of the pressure pulse thus contains high frequency components, in the neighborhood of 40 to 100 cycles per second—vibrations in the lower end of the audible sound spectrum. Propagated in the same way and at the same velocity as sound waves, these vibrations contribute to generation of the first heart sound but are beyond the frequency response range of clinical pressure-recording equipment. In brief, the first part of the pressure pulse can be heard but not seen.

The pressure pulse observed clinically begins with a steeply ascending limb in which a discontinuity is commonly observed. While the offset or discontinuity may be only a spurious vibration, it is tempting to speculate that it signifies a transition from one force to another within the inotropic phenomena of early systole. If this hypothesis is valid, identifiable forces in early systole are (1) the acceleration transient, and (2) the ejection pulse.

Acceleration transient. Peterson showed that an increment of flow added *very suddenly* to a fluid conduit results in an instantaneous pressure rise that momentarily far exceeds the immediately following steady state pressure appropriate to the new constant flow rate.[54] Moreover, the amplitude of the evanescent pressure peak is far in excess of that expected from the negligible volume added, and is only tenuously related to the expansile characteristics of the conduit. What is the clinical relevance of Peterson's acceleration transient?

During the isovolumetric phase of mechanical systole, pressure has developed rapidly within the ventricle. The aortic valve does not open, though, until the intracavitary pressure is somewhat in excess of the pressure at the aortic root. At the moment of valve opening the high energy state of the intracavitary fluid is abruptly communicated to the blood on the aortic side of the valve, imparting intense acceleration to this blood which had been at zero velocity (or even moving retrograde owing to coronary filling). The sudden translation of energy creates a steep-fronted, rapidly traveling wave disturbance. This "acceleration transient" (Peterson) is the force that initiates inscription of the upstroke of the pressure pulse.

Ejection pulse. The systolic upstroke is continued as a result of ejection of the first portion of the stroke volume into the aortic root. This produces distention of the aortic wall just distal to the valve and initiates a true pressure wave—a traveling disturbance that carries energy. However, pressure does not rise instantaneously throughout the vascular tree. Owing to the long column of fluid in the vascular tree that opposes global acceleration of the entire fluid mass, the pressure rise is initially confined to the most proximal segment of the aorta. The excess tension of the aortic wall in the first segment then displaces a very small amount of fluid into the next segment. This is accompanied by decline in pressure in the first segment and a rise in pressure in the second. Pressure is transferred in serial fashion distally from segment to segment; there is negligible net forward movement of the contained volume. A pressure wave has been initiated, and this wave will continue to travel rapidly toward the periphery even if there is no further emptying of the ventricle.

The upstroke of the pressure pulse is called the anacrotic rise ("up" plus "beat"). The duration of the upstroke is about 30 milliseconds. The anacrotic rise ceases rather abruptly, initiating the "shoulder" of the pressure pulse. With respect both to its steepness and to the peak that it obtains, the anacrotic rise of the pressure pulse is conditioned largely by the *rate of acceleration* of blood in the ascending aorta (as opposed to stroke volume, diastolic pressure, or aortic compliance). The rate of rise of the pressure pulse is related to the amount of sympathetic stimulation of the left ventricle.[56]

In summary, then, the initial portion of the pressure pulse is a qualitative indicator of myocardial contractility. It seems appropriate, therefore, to affix the label inotropic phase to the phenomena reflected in the early systolic inscription of the pressure pulse.*

Volume Displacement Phase

Were there no backup forces, the pressure pulse due to initial ejection would quickly fall away without significant displacement of blood toward the periphery. (This phenomenon is sometimes observed in a patient with a strong myocardium, intense peripheral vasoconstriction, and low cardiac output.) Normally, though, the more abrupt pressure-volume phenomenon is backed up, filled in, and sustained by continuing ejection of stroke volume from the ventricle. This is true flow rather than simply the development of pressure that follows modest volume displacement into an elastic chamber. Continuing volume ejection successively distends the partially collapsed aortic segments which lie in the wake of the early ejection pressure wave that has advanced at a more rapid rate toward the periphery. Pressure in the large vessels will be sustained or continue to rise inasmuch as pressure rises as long as flow into any vascular segment exceeds the volume of fluid leaving that segment. A notch in the pressure tracing (anacrotic notch?) may mark the discontinuity between the pressure pulse due to early ejection (inotropic component) and the more sustained volume displacement curve that follows.

---

*It is conceded that the rate of development of pressure cannot be equated unconditionally with inotropism inasmuch as the pressure-tension relationship is highly dependent upon the geometry of the heart. A very slight reduction in heart size permits attainment of the same pressure at much reduced wall tension. For authoritative discussions, see Braunwald and Sonnenblick and Strobeck.[7] [64]

The definitions of contractility and inotropism used in this text are presented in Chapter 1.

Thus there are commonly two peaks in the pressure pulse contour (Figures 3-1 and 3-2). The first is the inotropic component; the second, the volume displacement component. If the stroke volume is large relative to peripheral runoff during this period, then the second or volume displacement component of the pressure pulse determines the systolic pressure maximum. Under other circumstances, however, the observed maximum of the pressure pulse may be inscribed by the earlier peak of the inotropic component. As will be described later, the dual peak situation is of significance relative to the manner in which hydraulic couplings between subject and machine may modify these components, and with respect to the manner in which the readout device may be programmed to select or "see" a peak systolic pressure.

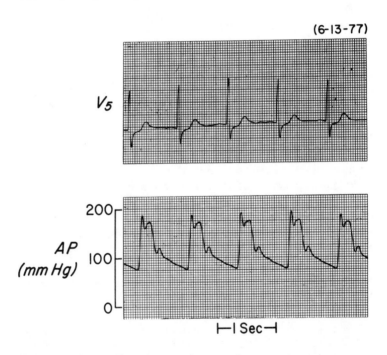

Figure 3-2 Two peaks are commonly observed in the pressure pulse at the periphery. Either may determine peak systolic pressure. Inotropic component is the higher in this example.
Radial artery cannula. Underdamped recording system. Resonant frequency about 20 Hz.

Late Systole and into Diastole

As ventricular emptying draws to a close, acceleration of flow assumes a negative value, rate of runoff exceeds volume input to the aorta, and aortic root pressure declines. With valve closure actual reversal of flow occurs in the aortic root owing to coronary flow and distention of the sinuses of Valsalva. Sharp deceleration of flow is manifest as a pressure event by inscription of the dicrotic notch. (At the periphery, the dicrotic notch is an artifact of reflection. This will be described later.) A prolonged, ramplike decline in pressure continues through diastole to the beginning of the next systole. The diastolic ramp is not undisturbed, however; definite undulations can be perceived. These are due to resonant waves in the great vessels and to reflections of energy from the periphery.

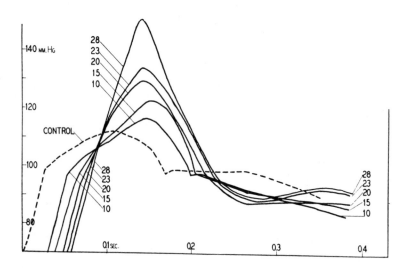

Figure 3-3 Increase in pressure pulse amplitude with increasing distance from aortic arch. Control (dotted line) is aortic arch tracing. Numbers on solid lines indicate distances down the aorta from the arch in dogs. "At its maximum in this experiment the pulse pressure exceeds that in the arch by more than 90 percent," but the mean pressures "are identical within the limits of error."[30]

Frequency response greater than 100 Hz is claimed for catheter and manometer system in this classic study. Reproduced with permission of the publisher, from: Hamilton, W.F., and Dow, P. *Am J Physiol.* 125:48–59, 1939.[30]

HOW THE PRESSURE PULSE CHANGES IN TRAVELING TO THE PERIPHERY

Things happen to the pressure pulse as it travels from the aortic root to the periphery. The several components become spaced out in time. Amplitude of some components is markedly augmented. Other components are damped or drop out. Finally, new elements are added to the pressure pulse that were not present at its genesis (Figure 3-3). Remington's description of the pressure pulse change is authoritative and precise: "The steep initial anacrotic rise remains unchanged in slope but persists for a longer time. Hence, the deflection marking its end, or the shoulder, comes at progressively higher pressure levels. The systolic peak becomes gradually narrower, so that the time from the start of the pulse to the peak is reduced..."[56]

Before describing how these changes come about it will be worthwhile to review the characteristics of the system with which we are dealing.

Teleologically, the purpose of the vascular tree is to accept hydraulic energy that is wholly pulsatile in nature and to transfer this energy to the periphery where it is dissipated as virtually continuous flow through viscous resistance. This performance requirement is satisfied largely by the capacitance (elasticity) provided in the structure of the major conduits. In operational terms the highly capacitive receiving system allows pulsatile emptying of the heart into a very low impedance. This means that the increase in pressure that follows a given increment of delivered volume is much less than it would be if the heart were required to empty into a nonelastic, purely resistive load. An element of inertance is introduced by the mass of blood that is accelerated and decelerated. Inertial effects, however, are much less prominent than those related to capacitance.

Any system containing capacitance and inertance will demonstrate certain characteristics. First, if excited, such a system will tend to continue to vibrate at a natural or resonant frequency specific for that combination of capacitance and inertance. Second, energy will be accepted by the system most easily when the frequency of delivered energy is the same as the natural frequency of the receiving or transmission system. Third, under these conditions there will be vigorous resonant oscillation within the system itself. (There are some frictional losses during oscillation, but oscillation itself does not dissipate energy.) Finally, flow and pressure are not in phase in an oscillating system.

All of the foregoing characteristics are evident in the arterial tree. The characteristics are greatly modified, though, by the complex anatomical structure of the system and because the pulsatile energy input to the system bears little resemblance to a simple sine wave defined by a single frequency. Physiologic investigation has not succeeded in delineating the weighting appropriate to these many factors in their complex combinations. However, qualitative recognition of these considerations is prerequisite to better appreciation of the changes wrought in the pressure pulse as it courses from aortic root to the periphery.

The first factor to be considered is resonance. Resonance *does* occur in the arterial tree. The resonant frequency varies from two to ten cycles per second. The higher resonant frequencies obtain in the presence of hypertension or increased cardiac output, while hypotension and low cardiac output are associated with lower resonant frequencies.[65] (For a bizarre example of resonance in vivo, see Figures 3-9 and 3-10.)

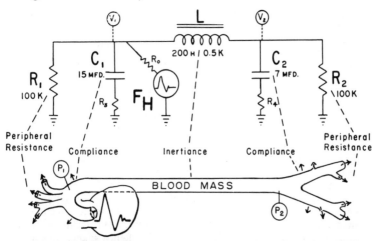

Figure 3-4 Electrical Analog of Systemic Arterial Tree, with Corresponding Anatomical Components.   When model is exercised, voltage waveforms measured at V_1 and V_2 closely resemble pressure pulses observed in vitro at sites P_1 and P_2. Reproduced, with permission of the publisher, from: Spencer, M.P. Pulsatile Flow in the Vascular System. Edited by W.F. Hamilton. In *Handbook of Physiology. Section 2: Circulation.* Vol. 2, Fig. 13. American Physiology Association. Baltimore: The Williams and Wilkins Co., 1963.[65]

The second consideration is that the systemic arterial tree cannot be simulated by a model depicting it as a single loop or circuit. Instead, the vascular tree behaves as though the heart were pumping into the bifurcation of two highly capacitive circuits connected in parallel (Figure 3-4). The aortic arch and the vessels to the head and upper extremities comprise one circuit, while downstream to an inductance (or inertance) are the abdominal aorta and lower extremity vessels which comprise a second capacitive circuit.*

This concept fits the observations that (1) pressures measured simultaneously in the upper and lower extremities are not in phase with each other, and (2) the lower extremity pressure (at least the systolic) is usually higher than that in the upper extremity. †

The parallel capacitance concept also fits the observation that occlusion or constriction of the aorta does *not* significantly increase the impedance at the input to the vascular tree unless the constriction is very close to the heart as in coarctation of the thoracic aorta. Moreover, the slightly different resonant frequencies of the two parallel capacitive circuits further insure that the input impedance is changed relatively little over a fairly wide range of frequencies brought about by marked changes in pulse rate.

The third factor to be considered is that the impedance of the arterial tree is not uniform. The systemic vascular tree is neither structurally nor dimensionally homogenous throughout its length.

---

*These are *not* functionally analogous to the dual circuits postulated by Caldini et al.[11]

† In measuring blood pressure, are the results dependent upon the techniques of measurement? Pascarelli and Bertrand found identical pressures in brachial and femoral arteries.[53] These were not really peripheral observation sites, however, in the context of characteristic impedance. It is of interest that their pressure curves were qualitatively dissimilar, the brachial tracing having a readily recognizable dicrotic notch, while the femoral did not. The tracings showed the expected time delay in onset of the femoral pulse relative to the brachial. Twenty-gauge needles coupled directly to the transducers were employed. Utilizing doppler ultrasonic technique, Felix et al. did find average leg systolic pressure to be slightly higher than average arm systolic pressure.[17] Bertrand and Pascarelli filed a rebuttal.[5] Johnstone and Greenhow, directly observing radial and dorsalis pedis pulses simultaneously, found the dorsalis pedis pulse arrived later and peaked higher (5 to 20 mm Hg) than the radial pulse.[37] (Their tracings, incidentally, show resonant waves at both sites, but no dicrotic offset in the pedal tracing.) Except for specifying 20-gauge catheters, the characteristics of their measuring system are not described.

It is a tapered tube rather than a cylinder of constant diameter; and the mix of elastic fibers and muscular elements is radically different in the smaller arteries as opposed to the aorta. As a consequence, each progressively more distal segment of the arterial tree appears to have an increasingly higher characteristic impedance. A substantial and abrupt increase in impedance occurs at the transition to the smaller arterioles, those of about one millimeter in internal diameter.

The gradually increasing impedance means that there will be a progressive increase in the amplitude of the pressure pulse as it travels distally. Thus, the height of the pressure wave really *is* greater in more peripheral vessels! Moreover, the opportunity for reflection is present at impedance discontinuities. Since the impedance changes are gradual and occur at multiple distributed sites, reflections are blurred and overlapping. The latter is not the case, however, at the periphery. Here the sudden discontinuity in impedance produces strong retrograde reflections of the pressure pulse, while pulse amplitude observed at a site close to the locus of reflection is greatly increased.*

A fourth consideration is the character of the pulse generated by cardiac ejection. This pulse is a non-sinusoidal phenomenon. Although most of its energy appears to lie in the range from 5 to 20 Hz (McDonald, 1960, cited by Strandness and Sumner), a broad spectrum of frequencies is generated up to and including those perceivable as sound.[68] It follows that this broad spectrum of frequencies may be acted upon in disparate ways by the highly nonhomogenous transmission system.

This expectation is realized in the fifth of this series of considerations: high frequency components of the pressure pulse travel faster than those of low frequency. Much as components of a mixture of compounds become progressively more separate in time as they pass through a gas chromatograph, so the components of the pressure

---

*The reactive impedance as well as the viscous resistance at the periphery are much greater than the impedance of the large elastic vessels. When the impedance at the input to a system is higher than the output impedance of the system driving it, there occurs (1) reflection of wave energy back into the driving system, and (2) an increase in the amplitude of the wave at the site of reflection owing to summing of the incident and reflected waves. See Chapter 1.

pulse exhibit "dispersion" with respect to time as they travel peripherally. The precise mechanism for dispersion is a subject of debate. Perhaps the differing frequency components may actually travel through differing, more congenial, media. The high frequencies near the audible spectrum, for example, may travel through the tense elastic walls of the vessel and not in the fluid per se. Low frequencies may travel in the form of momentary disturbances of the fluid medium: as true hydraulic pressure waves. The flow pulse—of very slow velocity—obviously involves forward movement of the blood itself. The term "dispersion" may be just another way of acknowledging that "phase shift" occurs in the elements of the pressure pulse as it travels peripherally in the tapered tube, with high frequency components coming to lead those of lower frequency. (The direction of this phase shift is just the reverse of that observed in transducer and tubing systems to be discussed later.)

Finally, high frequency components tend to disappear in transit. There are frictional losses owing to fluid viscosity and nonelastic walls. Moreover, it is characteristic of resonant systems that they accommodate frequencies rather well up to resonance, but beyond the resonant frequency the system response falls off more or less precipitously. (In the case of the arterial tree, inertance probably affords an increasingly important element of damping at higher frequencies.) Thus, the systemic arterial tree has been likened to a "low pass filter," one that preferentially accepts low frequencies, and has a resonant frequency below 10 Hz.[65]

In summary, the pressure pulse begins as a complex phenomenon and is subject to marked modification as it travels from the root of the aorta to the periphery. Broadly arched in its initial configuration, the pressure pulse increases in amplitude and becomes narrower as it travels. Its separate components show increasing temporal dispersion. Some elements disappear while other undulations are added as the energy package is processed through the systemic arterial tree. Reflection and pressure summation occur when the pressure pulse encounters abrupt impedance discontinuity at the periphery. The pressure effects of impedance discontinuity will be the object of further scrutiny in the next section.

ALTERATION OF THE PRESSURE PULSE BY RECORDING (OBSERVATION) TECHNIQUES

Influences of the Connecting System Between Patient and Transducer

When a wave travels down a tube that is closed at its distal end by an immovable obstruction, no energy can be absorbed and the wave is reflected back toward its source. In operational terms, a transmission system of a certain characteristic impedance has been terminated by an infinite impedance. In the presence of extreme impedance mismatch, strong positive reflection of the incident wave occurs. At the moment of reflection the pressure of the reflected wave is added to the pressure of the incident wave. The instantaneous pressure is the sum of the two waves and twice the size of either. If the element that closed the tube were a pressure-sensing device with no give or elasticity, it would record an instantaneous pressure twice as high as that observed by a similar pressure-sensitive element placed in the *wall* of the tube some distance upstream.

Common clinical practice for the direct measurement of arterial pressure involves placing an 18-gauge cannula in the radial artery. This virtually occludes the artery either by direct mechanical obstruction, resulting spasm, or eventual clot. In short, the cannula behaves as a total obstruction to flow and to wave phenomena. Therefore, there will be augmentation by positive reflection where the pressure pulse impinges on the indwelling cannula. This means that the apparent amplitude of the pressure pulse may be sharply magnified by the very process of exiting the vascular tree and entering the transducer system.

This should not be interpreted as an argument that smaller cannulas are a panacea for correction of exuberant systolic pressure readings. Any decrease in peak pressure associated with smaller-bore cannulas will be due more to increased damping than to diminished occlusion of the vessel, since the cross section of the cannula must be a very small fraction, indeed, of that of the vessel before significant reflection is ablated.[38] Besides, a cannula in the wrist artery is geographically close to the locus of the physiologic vascular impedance mismatch or discontinuity that exists at the periphery. Summing of incident and reflected pressure wave obtains in *all* arteries close to the periphery, cannulated or not, owing to that physiologic impedance discontinuity. A cannula at the periphery tends to "see" an augmented pressure peak because the cannula is where it is—not necessarily because of its occlusive character.

The import of impedance mismatch, reflection, and pressure summation (credited to Wiggers) is impressively shown by Van Bergen and colleagues' observation of direct pressure in the brachial artery via a 15 gauge (!) needle, followed by occlusion of the artery immediately distal to the cannula: "*Invariably* this increase in peripheral resistance resulted in an elevation of the direct systolic pressure of 20 to 30 mm Hg."[70] (Emphasis mine.)*

Additional transformations follow, for the cannula is typically connected to a stopcock and then to a transducer via a length of tubing. The transducer has a small but finite capacitance,† and there is additional springiness in the tubing. Inertance is contributed by the column of fluid in the tubing. Possessing both inertance and capacitance, then, the transducer and its connections constitute a resonant system.

With a four-foot length of connecting tubing, the resonant frequency of this system is about 20 Hz, though a small bubble will reduce the resonant frequency to 8 or 10 Hz. The damping factor is about 0.1 to 0.26—grossly underdamped! Thus the system is resonant at low frequencies and is likely to augment frequencies that may well be components of the pressure pulse. Moreover, the significant underdamping means that the ringing at resonance may result in a 75% to 150% increase in apparent amplitude of an incoming frequency that is near the resonant frequency of the system. Even a frequency that is only half the resonant frequency will be amplified as much as 30%! It is only when frequencies are very low, less than a third of the resonant frequency, that the transducer will respond by indicating an amplitude roughly equal to the amplitude of the exciting wave.

---

*Van Bergen adds "It is of interest to note that the values of auscultatory systolic pressures did not vary under the two conditions."
†A Statham P23AA transducer has a volume displacement of 0.8 mm³ per 100 mm Hg pressure. The displacement of the Statham P23Db transducer is 0.04 mm³ per 100 mm Hg.

What does all this mean? It means that the hydraulic connecting system influences to a marked degree what is observed as blood pressure. Low frequency components in the pressure pulse are likely to be transduced with a fair degree of faithfulness. Higher frequency components, though, are markedly accentuated in amplitude. The spurious augmentation of amplitude is particularly likely to affect the high frequency elements comprising the inotropic portion of the pressure pulse. Similarly augmented would be phenomena of rapid deceleration as well as reflections within the vascular tree.

The fact that the resonant frequency of the connecting system is very close to major frequencies in the pressure pulse also means that the transducing system will exhibit significant phase lag relative to the pressure in the artery. The phase lag will increase with increasing frequency, and be less marked at very low frequencies. Phase lag is of no great clinical significance. Failure to recognize phase lag, however, can seriously compromise conclusions about time-related events if based on observation of the peripheral arterial pressure pulse.

The following factors *increase* the resonant *frequency* of a system (the magnitude of change is indicated in parentheses):*

increase in radius of the tubing (proportional);
reduction of capacitance: reduction of compliance of
    transducer, increased stiffness of tubing (as the square
    root);
lower density of fluid in the tubing (as the square root);
shorter length of tubing (as the square root).

The following factors *increase damping:*

increase in viscosity of the fluid (proportional);
decrease in radius of the tubing (as *the third power!*);
increase in length of the tubing (as the square root);
increase in capacitance of the system (as the square root).

Thus, by selecting a transducer with a smaller displacement volume (diminished capacitance), the resonant frequency of the system will be raised—hopefully beyond the range of frequencies upon which it operates. However, a decrease in capacitance also causes decrease in damping. Thus, the trade-off could result in a

---

*The formulas are shown in Chapter 1.

worsening rather than an improvement in spurious amplification of critical frequencies.

Our studies indicate that relatively little improvement in frequency response is obtained by changing to a transducer of smaller displacement. This suggests that most of the frequency limiting occurs in the connecting tubing. Shortening the connecting tubing to a quarter of its original length would double the resonant frequency. Omitting the tubing altogether raises the resonant frequency to 50 Hz. Unfortunately, omission of the connecting link is not a feasible expedient in most clinical circumstances.

As is well known, a bubble introduced into the system markedly changes the characteristics of the pressure pulse recording: the tracing is markedly damped. (The bubble constitutes a marked increase in capacitance, thus increasing the damping.) More to the point, however, is the fact that a significant increase in capacitance markedly lowers the resonant frequency of the system, and it will simply fail to respond to the input of energy at frequencies higher than the new resonant frequency. As a result of the system's lowered resonant frequency, the pressure pulse tracing loses more and more of its high frequency elements and may even be degraded to mere undulations about a mean.

Since a connecting catheter about a meter in length and having a certain characteristic resistance is terminated effectively by a transducer diaphragm which cannot absorb energy but must only reflect it back into the source, can there not occur oscillations in the transmission system owing to this gross impedance mismatch? The answer is yes, such oscillations could occur, but the frequency of oscillation would be on the order of 100 Hz or greater and of no practical concern in clinical observations where the frequency range of interest probably does not extend much beyond 20 Hz.[20]

Electromechanical Factors

The frequency response of commercially available resistance strain gauges extends from zero to more than 100 Hz, more than adequate for clinical purposes. Amplifiers are another matter.

The frequency response of amplifiers for pressure recording may be variable from model to model within the same brand, and some are quite limited in high frequency response. This is something of a surprise inasmuch as it was not difficult to design an amplifier with a flat frequency response from zero to 100 Hz even in the days of tube-type devices. The answer may lie in the marketplace: an amplifier with an extended flat frequency response will faithfully reproduce all the exuberant oscillations and noise possibly injected by the hydraulic connecting system. Such fidelity may not find favor with customers. The surprising enigma of the "low fi" amplifiers is examined at length in Chapter 5. Here it suffices to note that some amplifiers roll off or begin filtering as low as 12 or even 8 Hz, and consideration should be afforded the loss of frequencies that might contain information of interest.

Readouts and recorders will be discussed in Chapter 5, and it will be pointed out that only the oscilloscope, with the "bouncing ball" type of display, can be relied upon to reproduce faithfully the pressure signal fed into it by a quality amplifier. Direct writers of all types, unless very expensive and impeccably maintained, invariably have an element of frictional drag that blurs and attenuates high frequency components. The shift register display (see Chapter 5), though pleasing to the eye, is tailored and smoothed in appearance, probably owing to filtering and to signal-sampling rates too low to permit fidelity reproduction of the pressure signal presented by the amplifier.

CLINICAL SIGNIFICANCE OF CHANGES
IN THE PRESSURE PULSE

At our present imperfect state of knowledge, the clinical significance of changes in the pressure pulse cannot be predicted but only surmised.

For decades past, the vagaries of pressure measuring techniques have been recognized, calibrated, and controlled by conscientious investigators in the laboratory. At the bedside and in the operating room, however, a curious naîveté about equipment prevails. Even though frustration may be expressed that the observed numbers are "not right," there exists an enigmatic failure to take the next step: acknowledge that the system and the site of measurement in large part influence or even create the values observed.

In reports of clinical studies it is virtually unknown to find specified the frequency response, damping, and other pertinent performance characteristics of the pressure recording systems utilized.

Since mean pressure is only modestly affected by changes in systolic pressure, and since peripheral resistance is derived from mean pressure and from flow averaged over several heartbeats, clinical studies founded on these mean values are not drained of merit. Moreover, nearly all of the power transfer in the systemic circulation is mean or "d.c.;" only about one-tenth of the total power is pulsatile about the mean.[12][68] Not so in the pulmonary circuit.[49] Fortuitously, therefore, left ventricular work estimates derived from mean values are not wide of the mark. Yet, it may be well to reflect on the thought that conclusions erected from many clinical blood pressure studies may rest on shaky foundations.*

It is not so much that our clinical equipment is faulty; rather, our perception of what the equipment tells us is naïve. Until our faulty perception is first acknowledged and then remedied, systematic exploration of blood pressure changes under varying clinical conditions—a task not yet undertaken—will not be a fruitful enterprise.

As a therapeutic maneuver, change in peripheral resistance is easily accomplished; and change in resistance will, indeed, significantly affect the power demand on the heart. But even when the clinician has succeeded in optimizing peripheral resistance and cardiac output, these manipulations may not suffice to wring from a compromised myocardium the last few percentage points of efficiency required for survival. The cost of the *pulsatile* component of cardiac power promises to be the next frontier for study and therapeutic manipulation.

Recognizing that both the contour and the absolute values of the peripheral arterial pressure pulse are altered by a wide variety of factors other than flow, two caveats are offered: first, efforts to quantitate *flow* on the basis of the pressure pulse, particularly as the pulse is observed at the periphery, are doomed to failure. Second, extreme caution should be exercised in pontificating that an observed change in the pressure pulse is due exclusively to a particular mechanism.

---

*See trenchant quotation in Chapter 1 from Yanof. Milnor, discussing pulsatile blood flow offers measured review of power, vascular pertubations, systemic versus pulmonary characteristics, and other themes pertinent to this text.[50]

With this bleak preamble, and despite the caveats, this section reviews the pressure pulse components. The review is embroidered by speculation as to how each component might be affected by clinical phenomena in the light of (1) origins of the pulse energy, and (2) knowledge of the performance characteristics of the systemic vascular tree.

The views expressed are no more than educated guesses and should be regarded with skepticism. The predications await validation (or defeat) through systematic observation in the clinical arena.

Inotropic Phenomena

The upstroke of the pressure pulse reflects ventricular inotropism and is related to velocity of myocardial fiber shortening and to peak aortic blood flow acceleration. The quality and the absolute amplitude of the inotropic portion of the pressure pulse are substantially modified in transmission through the vascular tree, and particularly by the hydraulic connections to the recording system.

Ventricular performance or inotropism is modulated by three factors. First is the preload, the amount of stretch of the muscle immediately prior to the initiation of contraction. Increasing preload increases velocity of shortening. Second is the afterload, or the weight that the muscle is required to lift after initiation of contraction. Increasing the afterload slows the velocity of contraction as well as decreases shortening.* The final factor is the intrinsic contractile state of the myocardium which is influenced by metabolism, calcium, and particularly beta-adrenergic stimuli.

The absolute height of the inotropic segment is not necessarily related to stroke volume, but instead to the interplay between inotropism and peripheral impedance. Indeed, if correlations

---

*Preload and afterload are defined in terms of a laboratory preparation involving weights and an isolated piece of muscle. Caution must be exercised in transferring these concepts to the intact vascular system. The geometry of the ventricle is complex, and the force opposing contraction is not constant through the duration of systole. (See Afterload and Contractility in Chapter 1; and footnote this chapter, in Origins of the Pressure Pulse.)

between stroke volume and early peak systolic pressure are explored, I suspect they will be *in*verse in many cases. The reasons are several. First, an increase in peripheral resistance tends to be associated with decrease in stroke volume; but increase in peripheral resistance leading to an increase in mean aortic pressure will tend to raise the resonant frequency of the arterial tree, moving it closer to some of the frequencies intrinsic to the inotropic component of the pulse. This will increase the amplitude magnification of the inotropic segment of the pressure pulse as it travels peripherally (even though stroke volume may be reduced). Second, marked increases in peripheral resistance will augment the already marked impedance mismatch at the threshold to the peripheral viscous resistance, tending to enhance reflection further. The strong positive reflected wave will be added to the incident wave, and the sum of the two will be perceived by the recording system.* Finally, the frequency content of the inotropic pulse is close to the resonant frequency of the external hydraulic coupling system, so that marked overshoot of a strong systolic upstroke may be anticipated—regardless of stroke volume—for reasons discussed earlier in this chapter.

While I have just suggested that increased peripheral resistance may increase impedance mismatch (discontinuity) at the periphery, it should be emphasized that peripheral *reactive* impedance and peripheral *resistive* impedance in the systemic circuit are separate entities geographically and functionally. The first significant impedance discontinuity at the periphery is reactive and occurs at entry to arterioles of about one mm in internal diameter. These are less compliant than larger vessels but, in the aggregate, offer little viscous resistance. True peripheral resistance occurs farther downstream: in smaller precapillary arterioles.

Remember also, that the heart is a long distance upstream, buffered from impedance changes at the periphery thanks to the impedance-matching function of the aorta. The heart "sees" or "looks into" an impedance (to pulsatile flow) that is relatively constant despite impedance changes at the periphery. Thus peripheral

---

*Since the locus of reflection is close to the peripheral site of observation, the summing ordinarily occurs without perceptible time delay. I suspect, though, that some of the notching in the upstroke observed with high-frequency display systems may relate to a slight time delay in transit of the reflection from 1 mm vessels back to the larger artery utilized for observation.

resistance, i.e., the resistance to continuous flow, may undergo significant changes without associated change in the (pulsatile) impedance seen by the heart.[12] Stated another way, peripheral resistance may increase significantly without affecting the change in pressure that the heart must generate to eject a given volume.

The noninterdependence of peripheral resistance, on the one hand, versus reactive impedance and inotropy on the other, is suggested by the pressure pulse recordings in Figure 3-5 obtained from a severely cirrhotic patient. In cirrhosis high cardiac output is associated with low peripheral resistance (here in the presence of a strong inotropic component). While resistance could be manipulated with phenylephrine (Figure 3-5 B), affecting the contour of the volume displacement component, the inotropic component of the pressure pulse underwent relatively little change.

In summary, apparent increases in the early systolic component of the pressure pulse are due primarily to (1) increased *rate* of generation of pressure (i.e., increased aortic blood flow acceleration, inotropy), and (2) enhanced reflection and resonance. Further modification is effected by the mean tension in the vascular tree which determines whether it will support the transmission of high frequency wave components.

The inotropic component of the pressure pulse may decline or disappear altogether owing to a variety of mechanisms. First, there may be primary myocardial depression due to pathologic changes, or as the result of anesthetic or other drugs, or owing to blockage or withdrawal of intrinsic beta-adrenergic stimulation. Second, the heart that does not fill will not empty forcefully. Decreased venous return from whatever cause will thus diminish the forces that generate the inotropic component. Finally, at the perimeter of the system, forces that decrease peripheral resistance may (but not always) serve to decrease the impedance mismatch, inhibiting generation of reflections.

Volume Displacement Phase

The high velocity inotropic wave is not related to forward flow. Flow is related to the volume displacement component of the pressure pulse, a component that succeeds the inotropic element after a usually perceptible discontinuity. The amplitude and duration of the volume displacement component reflect a balance between (1) the volume and rate of ejectate, and (2) the rate of runoff to the periphery. Figure 3-5 shows alteration of the configuration of the volume displacement component, presumably owing to alteration in peripheral resistance as a result of drug infusion. In Figure 3-6, marked changes in contour occur during ventilation as the result of waxing and waning of inflow to the left ventricle.

Late Systole and Diastole

Aortic impedance is low. This means the aorta accepts large increases in pulsatile flow with relatively little increase in pressure. One would expect, therefore, that substantial increases in stroke volume are *not* necessarily associated with prominent increases in the *amplitude* of the volume displacement component. In other words, an increase in stroke volume may cause little change in peak systolic pressure. Rather, there tends to be a *prolongation* or a broadening of the volume displacement component of the pressure pulse. Thus in the presence of a small stroke volume, the overall contour of the tracing is narrow; the systolic peak is promptly followed by a precipitous downstroke that plunges to a level not very far above diastole. The diastolic component, therefore, appears more like a plateau than a ramp. With a larger stroke volume the peripheral pressure pulse assumes a broader configuration, and the beginning of the now ramplike diastolic component joins the systolic downstroke at a much higher level.

This is the logical point at which to introduce the *dicrotic notch.* At the periphery the dicrotic notch is not an indication of aortic valve closure. Instead, the notch which seems to terminate the systolic downstroke is probably a time-delayed reflection, from the lower extremities back into the observation site in an upper extremity, of the inotropic impulse that was associated with the initiation of systole. There is a relatively constant interval between the onset of systole which generates the inotropic component and the reflection of that component from the distal (caudal) reaches of the arterial tree back into a wrist artery. On the other hand, the duration of the volume displacement component is quite variable. The dicrotic notch—more specifically, the reflected inotropic wave—generally falls into the trailing, descending edge of the volume displacement

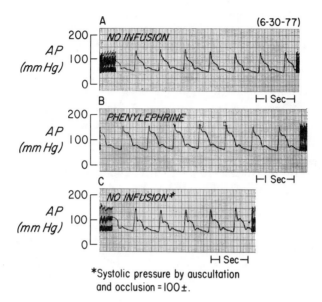

*Systolic pressure by auscultation
and occlusion = 100 ±.

Figure 3-5 Pressure Pulse in Advanced Cirrhosis A. The configuration of the volume displacement component is unlike the normal. Unmoderated obliquity of the downstroke suggests rapid peripheral runoff.
B. Administration of phenylephrine augments the volume displacement component, raising the mean pressure probably by decreasing runoff rather than increasing stroke volume. (Cardiac output determinations were not available.)
C. Five minutes after cessation of phenylephrine. Systolic pressure determinations by occlusion and by auscultation are found to correspond to peak of volume displacement component—50 mm less than the inotropic peak. What *is* this patient's systolic blood pressure? 150? 100?
In high output conditions such as cirrhosis, manipulation of blood pressure (as practiced here) in a seemingly hypotensive patient may not be beneficial unless possible reduction in total flow is associated with redistribution that actually improves perfusion to other presumably more vital areas. There are no data on this question.
A prominent inotropic component is not commonly observed in the presence of low blood pressure. Here it may reflect the hyperdynamic cardiac state associated with cirrhosis, permitted as long as the heart remains well-filled and competent.
Note low placement of the dicrotic notch.
Underdamped recording system. Resonant frequency: about 20 Hz. Radial artery cannula.

MGH   214 74 82 June 15, 1977

component. Therefore, the vertical location of the dicrotic notch will be a function of the duration or broadness of the volume ejection component. This accords with the clinical impression that a dicrotic notch high up on the pressure pulse curve is associated with a better flow state than if the notch is just a few millimeters above the lowest diastolic value, terminating a precipitous downstroke.

Under hypotensive conditions, the inotropic component disappears as does its delayed reflection, the dicrotic notch. The hypotensive pressure pulse, therefore, is not only low in amplitude but appears damped owing to the absence of sharp inflections.

As for diastole, a tracing that resembles an oblique ramp may be an indicator of substantial volume displacement toward the

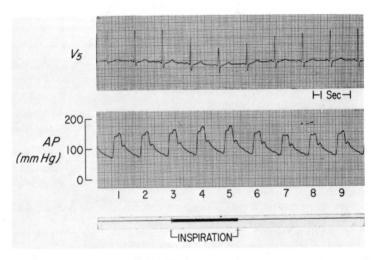

Figure 3-6 Respiratory Variation of Volume Displacement Component (Positive Pressure Ventilation). Initiation of positive airway pressure (third beat) shifts pulmonary blood volume. The result is augmentation of inflow to left ventricle, and increase in volume displacement component (fourth beat). Subsequent reduction of pressure on airway requires refilling of pulmonary system by right heart ejectate. This interval is associated with transient reduction of flow out of pulmonary circuit into left heart (sixth beat). Equilibrium is established near end expiration (beats seven, eight, nine), reflected in gradually rising volume displacement component.
Note shift in electrical axis associated with ventilation.
Underdamped recording system. Resonant frequency: about 20 Hz. Radial artery cannula.

MGH   June 8, 1977

periphery. In contrast, a relatively horizontal diastolic element suggests that little forward flow is occurring, the diastolic pressure level being maintained by high peripheral resistance.

The diastolic segment of the pressure pulse may be embroidered by oscillations owing to resonances in the arterial tree. A substantial dip in early diastole is to be expected in the presence of a well-filled vascular tree receiving substantial pulsatile input.

Manipulation of the Pressure Pulse

In summarizing the options for therapeutic intervention, one would think of propranolol as the drug to modify an exuberant inotropic component. If, on the other hand, mean blood pressure is low, and the problem is stunting of the later portion of the systolic trace, then one would think in terms of increasing venous return resorting to phenylephrine or by adding volume to the system.

Drugs that decrease arteriolar tone mimic the effects of exercise on the periphery. Arteriolar dilatation not only serves to decrease viscous peripheral resistance, but also diminishes somewhat the magnitude of the impedance mismatch at the periphery, thus favoring more effective forward transfer of energy accompanied by diminution of early systolic reflections that tend to exaggerate the apparent peak systolic pressure. Nitroprusside is regularly employed to reduce systemic pressure (Figure 3-7). This drug enhances the rate of runoff, so both the width and the height of the volume displacement component decline. While a decline in the inotropic component usually follows, on occasion it is necessary to add propranolol in order to effect pressure reduction. The logic of the treatment of hypertension, then, is dictated by which of the pressure peaks—the inotropic component or the volume displacement component—is the determinant of systolic pressure.

Halothane in low inspired concentration predictably effects reduction of systolic pressure after only a few minutes' administration. The effect is so rapid as to suggest that halothane works by shutting off exuberant sympathetic activity rather than by causing true cardiovascular depression.[26] The latter would imply significant tissue saturation which could be achieved only through using much higher inspired concentrations over a substantially longer period.[18] Enflurane may have effects similar to those of halothane, but is not as predictable. When halothane is administered in high concentration, its hypotensive effect may relate more to compromise of cardiac output than to reduction of peripheral resistance.

Pentolinium in doses of 1/100 those administered for controlled hypotension has proved effective in controlling perioperative hypertension, offering a practical substitute for halothane or nitroprusside. Though the appropriate flow studies have not been performed, it is conjectured that small doses of pentolinium damp ganglionically-mediated sympathetic stimulation. Larger doses of

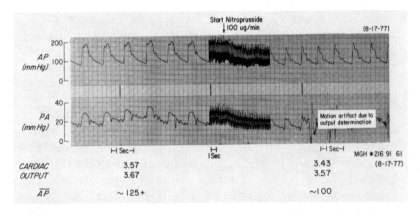

Figure 3-7 Change in Volume Displacement Component of Arterial Tracing by Vasodilator Therapy Change is dramatic with respect to height of volume displacement component; somewhat less with respect to width. (The changes were reversible within minutes of change in drug therapy and were readily reproducible.)
Note also:

1. The impedance discontinuity responsible for reflection of the inotropic component (and augmentation thereof) is largely unchanged.

2. Lowering of dicrotic notch without change in flow.

3. Mean pressure decreased. Flow was not changed (although left ventricular filling pressure decreased). Therefore cardiac power (work per unit of time) decreased.

4. Changes in dicrotic notch and changes in systolic components can be inferred from shading changes on slow-speed strip chart trace.

Cardiac outputs are in liters per minute, by thermodilution. Radial artery cannula. Underdamped recording systems. Resonant frequency about 20 Hz for arterial channel.

ganglionic blocking agents may produce hypotension primarily as a result of pooling in the venous side of the circulation, a form of exsanguination. The effect on perfusion is less beneficent, therefore, than if the same degree of hypotension were produced by nitroprusside which acts almost exclusively to reduce peripheral arteriolar resistance.

What about the load on the heart—the actual power output of the heart, and the fuel and oxygen cost of work per unit of time? The issues are complex, and the answers are not in. Factors to be considered are the complex impedances seen by the heart and the style in which the heart transfers energy into these impedances. As Jay Cohn puts it, we are "getting away from contractility" as the major determinant of cardiac function. Myocardial oxygen requirement may be conserved by asking the heart not to respond too rapidly.*

Changes in peripheral resistance do not change the impedance to pulsatile flow seen by the heart. This is because aortic input impedance is decoupled from peripheral resistance by the capacitance of the large elastic vessels. In other words, the left ventricle faces an almost constant oscillatory load, much smaller than the peripheral resistance, despite significant changes in that ("d.c.") resistance.[24] Thus, while isoproterenol reduces peripheral resistance, and angiotensin and norepinephrine increase peripheral resistance, aortic input impedance with respect to pulsatile flow is affected but little by such pharmocolgic interventions.[12]

This does not mean that systolic pressure will not be somewhat elevated when ejection is enhanced either as to velocity or volume. It merely means that the maximum pulsatile pressure change to achieve a given average flow can be much less than if the flow had to be delivered into a system of rigid pipes or directly through a fixed orifice (as in aortic stenosis).

The peak value of the brief inotropic component of the pressure pulse is subject to wide variation. (It sometimes reaches impressive heights during nitrous oxide-morphine-curare anesthesia.) Because of the brevity of this component, however, it contributes little to mean pressure. Inasmuch as perfusion is dependent on mean pressure, some might question the wisdom of trying to manipulate

---

*Lecture, Massachusetts General Hospital, November, 1975.

systolic pressure—especially if the observed absolute values of systolic pressure may in large part be artifacts of the recording system. Artifacts notwithstanding, the work of the heart is doubtless related to the *rate* of development of systolic pressure. Thus there may be merit in reducing early systolic values if this can be accomplished without compromise of mean perfusion pressure. One can strive by design and by trial pharmacologic intervention to strike an optimum balance between flow and the style of pressure generation in the patient with marginal cardiac resources.

It may transpire that drugs such as halothane and thiobarbiturates have been unfairly tainted with opprobrium as "depressors of cardiac function" (as evidenced by prolongation of the preejection period). Such drugs may in fact offer beneficent effects, analogous to the action of propranolol, in permitting the ventricle to achieve needed performance norms without excess energy expenditure.

The interplay of systolic forces and modifying factors is further suggested in Figure 3-8. The pressure tracings were observed during anesthesia for carotid endarterectomy wherein blood pressure was deliberately boosted during carotid occlusion. In the left panel in the figure, the myocardium is influenced by a powerful inotropic agent, yet the initial explosive systolic element in the pressure pulse tracing is not sustained by a significant volume displacement component. While the early and precipitous downstroke could be attributable to rapid runoff, the steep and ringing appearance of the preceding inotropic component suggests that the mechanisms for generation (of the spiky systolic pulse) are (1) reflection at the periphery, along with (2) exuberant amplification by the recording system—and that stroke volume is actually relatively small.

Later in the same case, halogenated anesthetic and inotropic drug were discontinued. Phenylephrine administration in very low dose was commenced. The pressure pulse assumed the configuration in the right panel of Figure 3-8. The initial inotropic component was much reduced. A broad volume displacement component appeared, and the dicrotic notch moved upward on the descending limb of the systolic curve. The second tracing suggests a healthier flow state.

It is simplistic to postulate a single mechanism for the salubrious effects of a particular drug such as phenylephrine on the pressure pulse under differing circumstances. In the example in Figure 3-8, the effect of phenylephrine was attributed to increase in mean systemic pressure* owing to increased tone in venous capacitance vessels, or redistribution of flow through parallel circuits with shorter time constants.[11][29] Through either mechanism (they are not mutually exclusive), venous return is increased, and increased stroke output follows. In the example of the patient with cirrhosis (Figure 3-5), on the other hand, it was postulated that phenylephrine increased peripheral arteriolar resistance.

Thus a drug may operate in different ways and through different mechanisms, given different starting conditions. This view is supported by some laboratory data and a host of circumstantial clinical evidence. In neither of the clinical cases discussed in the previous paragraph, however, was cardiac output determined (since placement of a thermodilution catheter was not warranted for the patient's benefit). Lacking this key measurement the postulated mechanisms of drug action remain speculative. Clinical studies to support or negate the proffered hypotheses are solicited in order to

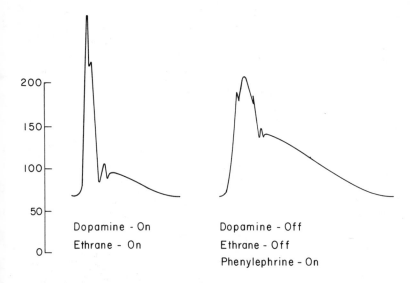

Figure 3-8 Manipulation of Pressure Pulse by Drugs Underdamped system. Resonant frequency about 20 Hz. Radial artery cannula.

---

*Mean systemic pressure, Guyton's term, is not to be confused with mean arterial pressure. Mean circulatory pressure might be less ambiguous.

improve patient care through more intelligent use of drug intervention. (Ironically, appropriate investigations are not likely to come to early fruition in today's inhibitory climate regarding human studies.)

An extreme example of modification of the pressure pulse, in this instance by anatomic factors, is shown in Figure 3-9. Each mechanical systole produced a train of large-amplitude, low-frequency oscillations. The abnormality was not in the recording system, but in the patient who had a very large abdominal aortic aneurysm. When the aorta was exposed, the aneurysm could be observed to dilate after cardiac systole and then eject the contained blood volume back toward the head—to all appearances like that of a wave oscillating back and forth in a water mattress. While occlusion of each of the iliac vessels had no apparent effect on the contour of the pressure pulse, surgical occlusion of the aorta just below the renal arteries dramatically established the relatively normal pressure pulse contour shown in Figure 3-10. It is significant also that surgical occlusion of the distal aorta does not usually produce an immediate marked increase in systolic pressure (since the major capacitance of the arterial system is distributed more proximal to the ventricle). In other words, even though peripheral vascular resistance may be increased by abdominal aortic cross-clamping, aortic input impedance is not dramatically changed.*

SUMMARY

The timing or phase relation, the frequency content, and the velocity of travel are quite different for each of the phenomena that inscribe the pressure pulse generated by mechanical systole. The components of the pressure pulse undergo dispersion as well as changes in amplitude in traveling to the periphery. Abrupt impedance discontinuity exists at the periphery. Reflection and

---

*Pressure rise does occur with cross clamping, but is neither instantaneous nor spectacular. The rise occurs because venous return to the heart continues almost unchanged for a few seconds after aortic occlusion, maintaining essentially the same cardiac output in the face of increased peripheral resistance.

resonance effect further inflections, waves, and amplitude changes in the pressure pulse.

Much altered from its form at the aortic root, the pressure pulse at the periphery is subjected to marked further modification when the external coupling system is underdamped and, at the same time,

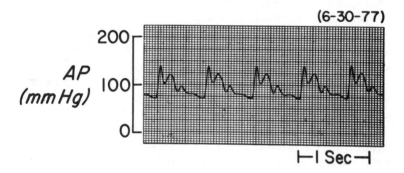

Figure 3-9 Peripheral Pulse Tracing from Patient with Large Abdominal Aortic Aneurysm Radial cannula, 18-gauge. Underdamped recording system. Resonant frequency about 20 Hz.

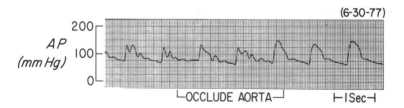

Figure 3-10 Change in Pressure Pulse Effected by Aortic Cross-clamping in Patient with Large Abdominal Aortic Aneurysm Iliac arteries had already been occluded without overt change in radial pressure pulse configuration. After aortic cross-clamping, diastolic pressure is the same and mean arterial pressure appears changed but little.
18-gauge radial artery cannula. Underdamped recording system. Resonant frequency about 20 Hz.

has an intrinsic resonant frequency close to that of the higher frequency components of the pressure pulse. Amplifier characteristics as well as those of the display system influence still further the tracing or numbers served up to the observer.

While the inotropic component and the volume displacement component of the pressure pulse are quite dissimilar in origin and significance, either—depending on circumstances—may determine the peak observed systolic pressure.

Drugs, respiration, and global changes in circulation markedly affect the character of the pressure pulse. In interpreting the significance of changes in the pressure pulse, however, it is important to keep in mind that the decoupling function of the great vessels insures that the impedance seen by the heart is relatively constant despite marked changes in impedance at the periphery.

I have refrained from applying the term distortion to changes wrought on the pressure pulse, for what happens to the pressure pulse—at least up to our cannula—is really a narrative of how the natural system performs. From the cannula outward, though, our contrivances may truly distort the physiologic signal. How significant this distortion may be in the guiding of therapy is imponderable at this writing. It is appropriate, though, to regard with enlightened skepticism the perceived numbers and waves, and to be both cautious and humble in drawing conclusions and in manufacturing presumptively therapeutic interventions.

In Chapter 1, discussing tides and estuaries, I pointed out that a common force may produce quite different effects according to dynamic modifiers operating in various parts of a global system. In our clinical observations of blood pressure at the periphery we are not unlike the visitor from outer space who naîvely draws inferences about terrestrial ocean tides while confined to a single vantage point at the landward end of the Bay of Fundy.

4 Blood Pressure: What Do the Several Measurement Methods Measure?

WHY MEASURE THE BLOOD PRESSURE?

Ritual produces a standard sequence of events without the necessity of reasoning. It is responsible for predictable uniformity and for easing the minds of participants trained in similar traditions. It confers power on the performer and grace on the recipient.

Editorial, *New England Journal of Medicine*[45]

Avoid hypotension and hypoxia.
Medical consultation.

Inferences about flow drawn from observations of pressure are permissible only if resistance is constant. The occasion to make valid inferences occurs rarely in clinical practice since the preferred *modus operandi* of the body's wisdom is to effect required changes in perfusion by altering resistance rather than pressure. This is true over a broad range of flows and under conditions pathologic as well as physiologic.

Control of perfusion is largely automatic because regional vascular resistance is regulated by local metabolic requirements. In turn, regional alterations of peripheral resistance markedly affect return flow and cardiac filling pressure, particularly if there is redistribution of flow through parallel channels of differing capacitance.[11] Venous return determines cardiac output since the competent heart merely pumps out that which is fed into it.[28][29]* Thus there exists an autoregulatory mechanism in which total flow is manipulated in order to maintain constant systemic pressure despite marked changes in resistance.

Consider, for example, arteriovenous shunting. Whether localized or distributed (as in the case of cirrhosis), shunting is associated with cardiac output greatly in excess of normal but without significant abnormality in mean arterial pressure. If it is possible surgically to close a significant arteriovenous fistula, effecting marked increase in peripheral resistance, then heart rate and ventricular filling pressure change dramatically—but there is little alteration in blood pressure as flow is reduced to the normal range.

The other extreme of resistance manipulation is observed in diving mammals. During submersion peripheral circulation is virtually shut off and the animal shifts to anaerobic metabolism even in those muscles actively being exercised in the pursuit of prey. This dramatic alteration in flow is associated with remarkably little change in mean arterial pressure, presumably to protect the cerebral circulation from extreme overpressure.[61][57][16]

Gross qualitative inferences perhaps may be drawn from changes in blood pressure, and it has been speculated elsewhere in this text that the configuration of the pressure pulse may contain information bearing on *how* the pressure is generated. The latter may have more pertinence to the cost of work performed by the heart than does the actual pressure attained. Moreover, anesthesia

---

*Even complete denervation of the heart hardly affects the ability to regulate cardiac output.

commonly involves administration of drugs that depress myocardial contractility and at the same time diminish peripheral resistance. It may be allowed, therefore, that pressure measurement is not wholly devoid of merit, and that there are occasions when low blood pressure *does* have positive correlation with low flow.

Not warranted, though, is the assumption that low blood pressure is necessarily bad.* Controlled hypotension is regularly induced in the operating room and has proved remarkably free of cerebrovascular, cardiac, or renal problems even in patients of advanced age. The presumption is that organ perfusion remains adequate owing to the mechanisms utilized to induce the hypotension. As the renologist Normal Hollenberg puts it, "It's not so much the blood pressure but the way the kidney reacts to it."

If blood pressure evaluation is such a dubious exercise, why do it at all? The question is valid; much of what we do is the exercise of ritual. One saving grace: the ritual forces us to observe the patient and sometimes even touch him. It is suggested that this is a salutary exercise that should not be abdicated to machinery any more than is necessary. Little merit is seen, though, in recording blood pressure more closely than the nearest five or ten millimeters of mercury. More meticulous recording suggests the observer is taking the ritual too seriously and is naive regarding the vagaries of the process.

Since blood pressure tells little about flow, why be concerned with what the various techniques measure? The main answer is that the motivation for this text was repeated exposure to concerns that those caring for sick patients regularly harbor, and oft express with asperity, regarding disparities encountered when the blood pressure of the same patient is measured by different methods. Achieving understanding of what is observed may allow better appreciation of why discrepancies exist.

A second answer is that, in measuring blood pressure, we are dealing with a variety of artifacts. These artifacts are but tenuously related to the physiologic processes that we really would like to know about—processes such as regional perfusion and metabolic needs. Yet, appreciation of the composition, foibles, and sometimes

---

*It is equally naive to assume that a high blood pressure means that things are good.

misleading dimensions of these artifacts may lead us more closely to a better understanding of what is really going on with our patients.

Still another answer is that we can't compare measurements unless we all use the same measuring sticks. At the very least we must be aware of the need to calibrate the operating discrepancies between your system and mine. If the measurement errors turn out to be quantitatively similar, or if reasonable conversions are permissible, then we will be in a better position to accumulate and exchange information aimed at improving the care of future patients. The numbers may still not be "right," but at least we operate from—as the jargon puts it—"a common data base."

Finally, even though numbers between systems are not necessarily comparable, and the blood pressure may be only a relative index of true pressure (which will not be defined in this book), some systems may indeed be more useful than others in diagnosis or guidance of therapy. Moreover, the relative utility of a given system may vary according to time, patient imperatives, convenience, clinical need, and economic reality.

The following sections set forth analyses of several techniques of blood pressure measurement. While based in part on reviewed literature, the analyses are embroidered with frankly editorial views stemming from prolonged observation of patients subject to trauma, infection, and major vascular manipulation—surgical as well as pharmacologic. Studies available from the past bear conclusions often vague and conflicting; nor are past studies necessarily pertinent either to (1) the classes of patients we now manage, or (2) the clinical measurement systems in common use in the 1970s. There are no systematic studies of patients subject to manipulation by cold, vasoactive and inotropic agents, and major occlusions of the aorta. If and when such patients are systematically observed, reports of data should incorporate regard for modifiers operating (a) in the vascular system, (b) at the measurement system interface with the patient, and (c) in the measurement system itself.

While the descriptions of noninvasive and composite measurement techniques are referenced to direct measurement via a peripheral arterial cannula, the analysis of the pressure pulse in Chapter 3 indicates that directly measured blood pressure is per se a process wrought with vagaries, inconsistencies, and unknowns. It may be expedient to utilize directly measured blood pressure as a reference; but to regard the direct (or any other clinical blood pressure measurement technique) as accurate, right, or the ark of gospel, borders on the foolhardy.

THE RIVA-ROCCI (AUSCULTATORY) METHOD

Flow that is otherwise laminar is rendered turbulent in passing through an orifice. Turbulence means that sharply localized pressure gradients or cells of inhomogeniety exist within the fluid. Inhomogenieties within a medium can be detected by a variety of means. If the cells of turbulence within a blood vessel or heart chamber are generated at a rate corresponding to the frequency of audible sound and contain sufficient energy, even a device as crude as a stethoscope can be utilized to detect them.

Flow in major arteries is largely laminar but can be rendered turbulent owing to luminal irregularities or as a result of vascular deformation by force applied from the outside. Application of external pressure to produce deformation of the brachial artery is the principle involved in the auscultatory technique of blood pressure measurement. When a pneumatic cuff of proper dimensions is applied to the upper arm and inflated to a pressure exceeding systolic pressure, the artery is compressed to occlusion. Since there is no flow, no sound will be detected through a stethoscope placed just distal to the cuff. As the cuff is deflated to a pressure just below that of systole, with each heartbeat there will be a slight squirt of turbulent flow issuing from the artery distal to the cuff. Acoustically detected and related to the air pressure within the cuff, the onset of this turbulence denotes systolic pressure.

As the cuff is further deflated the compressed artery will be permitted to eject blood for progressively longer portions of the interval between systole and diastole. Flow immediately distal to the cuff will still be turbulent and sounds continue detectable. Finally, as the cuff pressure reaches diastolic pressure, the artery is no longer occluded for any part of the interval between systole and diastole. Flow returns largely to laminar form and there is abrupt diminution of the sounds of turbulence. Some deformation of the artery continues until the cuff pressure is well below that of diastole, so some turbulent sounds may still be perceived. Therefore, an abrupt change in quality (muffling) of the sounds is considered to indicate the attainment of diastolic pressure.

The noises of turbulent flow are the Korotkoff sounds, and they have been studied in detail.* The foregoing description of their generation is practical but oversimplified, inasmuch as certain unusual conditions (such as aortic regurgitation) are associated with persistence of sounds to zero cuff pressure.[25]

Since the generation of Korotkoff sounds is wholly dependent on flow, but there may be pressure without flow, it follows that there will *not* be an inexorable correlation between central arterial pressure and the pressure determined by the auscultatory technique. Van Bergen and associates concluded from their extensive study that (1) indirect readings of blood pressure, diastolic as well as systolic, consistently fall below the direct measurement values, and (2) "the drift of indirect readings is to fall increasingly below the direct measurement as blood pressure increases."[70]

Our own observations† indicate that there is a fair (within 20 millimeters) correlation between the auscultatory systolic pressure and the peak value of the volume displacement component of the directly observed radial arterial pressure pulse. A rough correlation also exists with respect to diastolic values. Occasionally, however, pressure measured by cuff is substantially higher than that observed with direct measurement.‡ Perhaps this is due to diminished compliance of the brachial artery and surrounding tissues.

Conditions inhibiting flow will produce marked disparity between cuff pressures and direct pressures. Flow-inhibiting conditions are of two types: (1) primary reduction in cardiac output due to diminished venous return or to compromise of cardiac contractility, and (2) reduction of flow owing to increased peripheral resistance. The auscultatory technique may fail completely under extreme but not unusual conditions.

In the instance of deliberately induced hypotension, for example, not only is mean flow diminished but pulsatile flow is much less energetic. Blood pressure becomes undetectable by the auscultatory

---

*For an extensive account of Korotkoff sounds, frequency and energy content, detection, and historical references, see Whitcher in Bellville and Weaver and also McCutcheon et al.[46][74]

†Under uncontrolled working conditions. The systems were grossly underdamped (damping factor about 0.2), with resonant frequency approximately 20 Hz, varying from 11 to 28 Hz with conscientiousness of flushing.

‡For a report of dramatic disparity see Wallace et al.[71]

method even though intravascular pressure is sufficient to maintain excellent peripheral perfusion.

Reduction of flow due to increased peripheral resistance may be generalized or localized. A common example of the latter is infusion of cold fluid into the arm that is utilized for cuff pressure determination. As the arm and hand cool, cuff pressure seems to diminish and the Korotkoff sounds become increasingly difficult to hear. Central pressure may actually be unchanged. As for generalized peripheral vasoconstriction, this occurs with cold, hypovolemia, and with the administration of vasoactive drugs. The extreme case has been encountered with administration of norepinephrine: the extremities become cold and blue-white, peripheral pressures are unobtainable by cuff, yet directly measured arterial pressure is far in excess of normal.

DOPPLER METHODS

The pitch of the sound generated by a noisy airplane, train, or automobile is higher when the vehicle is moving toward you than when it is moving away from you. When the noisy vehicle passes at close range, there is a sudden downshift in the pitch of the sound. The effect of relative motion on the apparent frequency of wave phenomena was described in 1842 by Christian Johann Doppler, an Austrian mathematician and physicist. Combined with echo ranging, there was spirited development of applications of the Doppler principle during World War II to refine the sonar systems used in antisubmarine warfare.

Echo ranging is the measurement of the time delay of a reflected sound wave in order to determine the distance between the observer and the reflecting object. The *doppler effect,* on the other hand, is used to determine whether a reflecting object is moving toward or away from the observer, and at what relative speed. The echo ranging and doppler techniques use similar electromechanical apparatus. The differences are in the way the echo data are processed and displayed.

Both processes depend on the reflection of high frequency sound waves. A transducer emits a very short pulse of sound at a specific high frequency. The same transducer then serves as a microphone to listen for reflection of the sound wave pulse. When received, the reflected signal is analyzed either as to time delay, which gives distance information, or as to shift in frequency, the latter being a measure of the velocity of the reflecting target relative to the sound source. "Up doppler," or an increase in pitch, indicates the target is moving toward the observer, while "down doppler" indicates relative motion away from the observer.

Diagnostic ultrasonic laminography is a highly sophisticated application of echo ranging, while the doppler effect (frequency shift) is utilized in much simpler equipment for blood pressure measurement.

There are two types of doppler measurement of blood pressure. Both suffer from being least reliable when most needed. The types are (1) detection of flow within a vessel, and (2) detection of motion of the blood vessel wall. In each case, a pneumatic cuff coupled to a manometer serves to indicate the externally applied pressure at which an event occurs that can be detected by the doppler sensor.

Detection of axial flow in a small vessel distal to an occluding cuff would appear a simple, convenient, noninvasive tool in difficult situations such as blood pressure management in the small infant or in the severely burned patient. Unfortunately the doppler transducer is exquisitely position-sensitive and is prone to dislodgement by drapes or patient repositioning. When failure does occur it is not easy to determine whether the blood pressure or the measurement system failed. Moreover, the system becomes unusable in the presence of the electrosurgical instrument.

While axial flow detection provides only systolic pressure information (if the technique works at all), doppler detection of vessel wall *motion* will provide diastolic as well as systolic values. Again, the detector has proved highly vulnerable to modest agitation by the surgical team. The ensuing erratic readings limit applicability of the instrument in management of controlled hypotension. The device is cumbersome, defeated also by the electrosurgical unit, and the cost exceeds that of a quality two-channel conventional monitor.

It has been suggested that the automatic doppler device might be useful in the management of the patient with a thoracic aortic aneurysm when it is considered desirable to lower blood pressure artificially but postpone invasive observation.

OSCILLOTONOMETRY

The Oscillotonometer

Geddes has reviewed the rise and present eclipse of oscillotonometry.[21] The relationship of values obtained with this technique compared to those obtained with the auscultatory technique can charitably be described as elastic if not tenuous. The comparative values generally change in the same direction at the same time, but a concordance more precise than tens of millimeters of mercury is not to be expected. Variances are owed in part to an absence of uniformity of opinion regarding what degree and quality of oscillation of the needle denotes systole and diastole, and also to the highly subjective nature of such end-point criteria. Literature supplied by the importer of the oscillotonometer states that systole is indicated when feeble and regular excursions of the pointer "sharply increase in value and become erratic" as air is bled via the valve on the body of the device. Maximum excursion of the dial pointer in the sensitive mode probably occurs about 20 millimeters below systolic pressure.[21]

However dubious the accuracy of the numbers, an advantage of the oscillotonometer is that readings can be obtained even when pressure is too low, or flow too poor, to permit utilization of the auscultatory method. Thus the oscillotonometer is favored by some for management of controlled hypotension.

The oscillotonometer is not a simple instrument. Combined in a single ingenious mechanism are (1) a tonometer which indicates pressure relative to atmospheric, and (2) an oscillometer or sensitive plethysmograph. A better appreciation of what this instrument does may be afforded by examination of how it works.

The oscillotonometer utilizes parallel inflatable bladders or cuffs held in a fabric jacket encircling the arm (so that the bladders are at a right angle to the axis of the humerus). The pressure cuff is quite narrow compared to the width considered optimum for appropriate recognition of systolic pressure utilizing the Riva-Rocci technique. The airtight case of the instrument (Figure 4-1) houses two pressure-sensitive (anaeroid) wafers: the pressure wafer (6 in the figure), and the oscillometric or sensitive wafer (11 in the figure). The pressure wafer is similar to the element in an ordinary anaeroid manometer and will tolerate pressures up to 300 mm Hg; it differs in

92

(Reproduced with permission from the publisher, from: Instruction Pamphlet. Propper Manufacturing Co., Inc. 36-04 Skillman Ave., Long Island City, New York 11101.)

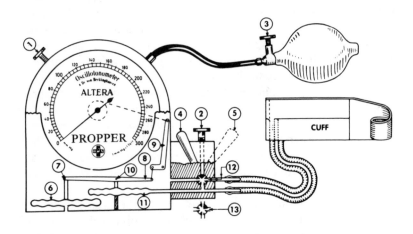

Figure 4-1   Oscillotonometer (Slightly Modified)
1 Zero adjust.
2 Bleed valve adjustment screw.
3 Bulb pressure release valve.
4 Control valve lever: normal position, read pressure.
5 Control valve lever: position to bleed, observe oscillometry.
6 Pressure wafer.
7, 10, 8 Pivot points on internal lever.
9 Bell crank.
11 Sensitive oscillometric wafer.
12 Connection port to valve rotor shown in pressure or normal position (control lever in position 4).
13 Position of valve rotor to bleed, observe oscillometry.

that the interior of the wafer communicates freely with the atmosphere, while the exterior is exposed to the pressure within the instrument case. As for the oscillometric or sensitive wafer, it is very compliant and its interior is always directly connected to the distal of the two cuffs. Each wafer is fixed to the wall of the case by a rigid post. The opposite face of each wafer is pivoted to separate points on a common lever that activates the dial pointer via a bell crank **9** and chain.

Compression of the hand bulb forces air into the sealed case and thence into each cuff simultaneously. Manual compression is continued until the indicated pressure, the same in both cuffs, is well above the anticipated systolic pressure. Note that the pressure inside the sensitive oscillometric wafer **11** is the same as the pressure in the case surrounding the wafer, so the wafer does not change in volume. Its pivot **10** thus serves as the fulcrum for the internal lever (**7, 10, 8**), of which the force arm (**7, 10**) is displaced in proportion to the differential pressure across the pressure wafer. The pointer indicates the pressure in the case and in the two cuffs.

Manual shifting of the spring-loaded control lever (from position **4** to **5**) aligns the bores in the valve as indicated in inset **13**. This permits *slow* loss of air via bleed valve **2**, from the case, from both cuffs, and from the interior of the sensitive wafer. As pulsatile blood flow begins to escape under the proximal cuff, oscillating volume changes occur in the distal cuff. These volume changes are transmitted unobstructed to the interior of the sensitive oscillometric wafer and create small pressure changes within it. The sensitive wafer is free to expand and contract with each pulse because the case pressure represents a slowly declining mean, averaged over several beats, while the pressure *inside* the sensitive wafer oscillates about this mean with each heartbeat. As for the pressure wafer, its volume changes very little during this operation, so that its pivot **7** to the internal lever now becomes the fulcrum of that lever while pulsatile operating force is applied via the pivot **10** of the sensitive wafer. The latter's effect on the pointer is exaggerated by this change in class of lever operation.

When sharp oscillations of the pointer are first observed during the bleed operation, the control lever is permitted to snap back to its original position **4**. The pressure in the case now is the same as that in the proximal cuff. Although small damped oscillations of pressure continue in the system, the important consideration is that pressure fluctuations in the case are now equal to, and in phase with, any pulsatile pressure changes inside the sensitive wafer. Sensing no differential pressure, the sensitive wafer ceases to oscillate. Its now stable pivot reverts to being the fulcrum for the internal lever, while the force arm of the lever is again operated by deformation of the pressure wafer. The pointer indication at this juncture is taken as the systolic pressure.

The choice of end point indicating *diastolic* pressure is subject to somewhat murky debate, but the mechanical process controlling the needle movement can be deduced from the foregoing operational description.

"Flicker" Method

The "flicker" technique might be called the poor man's oscillotonometry. It utilizes only a conventional blood pressure cuff and a standard aneroid manometer. As the cuff is slowly deflated, the meter needle begins to jump in cadence with the heartbeat. As the cuff pressure is lowered still further, the needle begins more regular oscillation of greater amplitude so that the upward and downward excursions are approximately equal.

Although our data have not been subjected to statistical evaluation, in a series of more than one hundred observations it was found that the point of maximum oscillation of the needle corresponds remarkably well with the systolic pressure as determined by the occlusion technique (to be described shortly in this chapter).* The concordance is usually within 30 millimeters, often within 20 or even 10 millimeters! Reasonable concordance and readability were maintained even though patient temperatures dropped as low as 33 °C during protracted surgery.

Problems with this technique include the highly subjective nature of the end point and the fact that only systolic pressures are indicated. Nonetheless, the method may not be wholly without merit in following trends or in supporting observations from other techniques.

DIRECT OR INVASIVE PRESSURE MONITORING

The intricacies of direct arterial pressure measurement are primarily described in Chapter 3, concerned with devolution of the pressure pulse, and in Chapter 5 which deals with methodology.

---

*Bruner, J.M.R., Krenis, L.J. and Kunsman, J.M., unpublished observations, 1977.

Measurement in Peripheral—and Not so Peripheral—Arteries

Radial or ulnar arteries are customary invasion sites, and relatively large bore cannulas are utilized (18-gauge). On occasion—for expediency or diagnosis—pressures may be observed elsewhere, and factors that alter the quality as well as absolute amplitude of the tracing must be kept in mind. For example, Figure 4-2 shows tracings obtained almost simultaneously from the radial and the carotid arteries in the same patient. The same transducer was used, connected in each case to tubing of identical type and length. The carotid, however, was entered with a 22-gauge 1½″ needle, while an 18-gauge cannula lay in the radial artery.

In the carotid tracing some damping is doubtless owed to the smaller bore needle. The excursion of the pressure pulse in the carotid, however, probably *is* of lower amplitude and more extended than the pressure at the radial cannula site. This is because the carotid needle resides in an area of lower characteristic impedance so there is less amplification of the pressure pulse. Moreover, the needle neither occludes the artery nor is there immediate distal occlusion, so reflection augmentation of the pressure pulse is minimal. Similar considerations would apply in assessment of the pressure pulse obtained from the femoral artery. In addition, even greater phase lag would be anticipated at the more distal site.

The Occlusion Technique

This is a composite technique. It utilizes a pneumatic cuff connected to a mercury or aneroid manometer plus observation of the arterial pressure pulse via an inlying cannula. Two observers are usually required: one manipulates the pneumatic cuff and watches the manometer as the cuff pressure is slowly reduced from a value above systolic; the other observer, watching the oscilloscope screen, calls out when the first pip appears on the otherwise flat line, signifying that arterial flow is escaping under the pneumatic cuff. The height of the mercury in the manometer at this point is taken as the systolic pressure.

We have found that systolic pressures determined in this manner correlate fairly well with the second peak—the volume displacement component—of the directly displayed arterial pressure pulse.

96

Similarly, there is reasonable correlation with systolic pressure as determined by the Riva-Rocci method.*

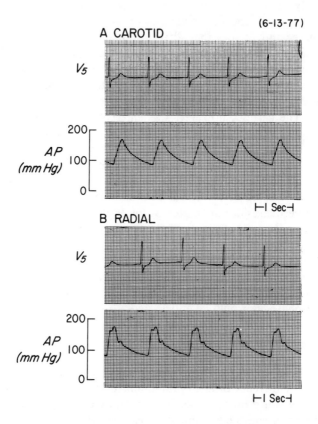

Figure 4-2 Carotid Compared to Radial Pressure Pulse Save for 1½ " 22-gauge needle in carotid vs 18-gauge 2 " cannula in radial artery, recording systems are identical (same transducer and same length of connecting tubing). Onset of upstroke after Q is 0.20 seconds in radial, 0.16 seconds in carotid. Though dicrotic notch is damped in carotid, note that in each tracing the notch follows about 0.28 seconds after the start of the systolic upstroke.

---

*Bruner, J.M.R., Krenis, L.J. and Kunsman, J.M., unpublished data, 1977.

The occlusion technique does not require that the direct pressure monitor be calibrated. (Indeed, no electronics are required: a bubble in the cannula's connecting tubing will serve as a pulse detector.) However, it does not follow that the electronic monitor should be calibrated to agree with systolic pressure observed by the occlusion technique. Commonly noted, this practice is to be deplored. There are a multitude of reasons why the air pressure in the occluding cuff is likely to be different from the systolic pressure displayed by the electronic monitor. A major reason, alluded to repeatedly in this text, is the fact that the ostensible peak systolic pressure may be determined by either of the two systolic peaks found in the pressure pulse tracing. The second peak is presumed to be a flow phenomenon, while the first is probably a true pressure wave that may not be transmitted through the occluding cuff.

In support of the foregoing, try this experiment: hold taut a piece of clothesline attached to a springy post set in the ground some distance away. Shake your arm up and down, and you will create waves that run along the rope to the post. By pulling on the rope you can displace the top of the post toward you; with release of tension on the rope, the post springs back.

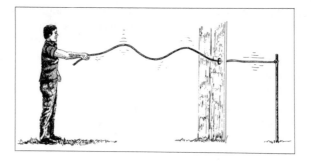

Figure 4-3 **An Experiment to Show Why Occlusion Pressure is Usually Lower Than Directly Measured Systolic Pressure** Wave motion, but not axial displacement, is inhibited by constraint upon motion perpendicular to the longitudinal axis of the medium (a rope, in this case).

Repeat the experiment, but this time put the post in your neighbor's yard and run the rope through a knothole in the fence between your properties (as shown in Figure 4-3). By alternately tugging and releasing the rope, you can still produce significant displacement of the top of the post; but when you try to make waves, the waves travel only as far as the knothole and do not proceed to the post. The knothole damps wave motion along the rope but does not inhibit axial displacement.

Insofar as the components of the pressure pulse are concerned, the compressing cuff on the upper arm acts like the knothole in your neighbor's fence. Even though axial displacement (flow) is permitted, traveling (pressure) waves are almost completely blocked.

Nonelectrical Methods for Direct Measurement of Pressure

Blood pressures were measured directly and recorded before the age of the electron. A simple mercury-filled U-tube from the physics laboratory serves quite well as an indicator of mean pressure. Inertia of the mercury column precludes delineation of systolic and diastolic pressures.

An aneroid manometer may be similarly used. It is connected to the indwelling cannula by a length of tubing containing an air buffer. The length of the air column has no effect on the accuracy of the indicated pressure. If this technique is used, it is essential that the aneroid manometer be protected from transgression by fluids or blood. This can be assured by keeping the manometer at least several inches above the air-fluid interface, or interposing a compliant membrane barrier (commercially available) between patient and manometer. The manometer is not to be attached to the patient's armboard or cutely cradled in his hand; this pernicious practice regularly allows fluid and blood to enter the manometer. Even if the expensive device is not ruined, the next patient is exposed to the risk of infection from the contaminated manometer.

MEAN PRESSURE

The commonly used formula for mean pressure is wrong. Mean pressure is not the diastolic pressure plus one-third of the pulse pressure. Mean pressure is the time-weighted average of a series of instantaneous pressures.[68]

Compare the two panels in Figure 3-8. Calculated by the conventional formula, the mean pressure of the tracing in the left panel would be higher than that in the right. Yet the area under the curve in the right panel is much greater than in the left. A true mean pressure, graphically or electrically determined* for the tracing on the left, would be quite different from the formula mean. So might conclusions of therapeutic import drawn on the basis of means conjured up by different modes of computation.

---

*Only a simple electronic circuit is required to provide the mean of an undulating signal.

5 Invasive Pressure Monitoring

PRESSURE MONITORS

A pressure measuring system has the same components as a home music system (Figure 5-1): an input transducer, a package of electronic elements, and an output transducer.

The phonograph cartridge of the music system converts weak mechanical energy into a small electrical signal. The preamplifier augments the electrical signal and filters and conditions it if

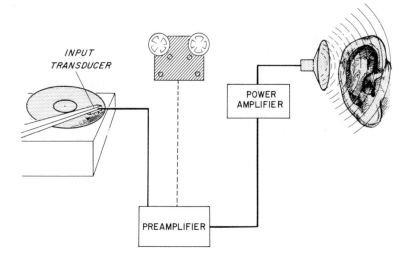

Figure 5-1 A pressure monitor has the same components as a music reproducing system.

necessary. Most of the user-operated controls are found on the preamplifier. A power amplifier further strengthens the signal to drive the output transducer. For music this is a loudspeaker, but the output transducer or readout can be a cathode ray tube or any other device that converts an electrical signal into some form that may be appreciated by a receptive intellect.

At some stage in the electronics, the electrical signal may be picked off and fed into an information storage device such as a tape recorder. From here a facsimile of the analog signal can be retrieved for reexamination at a convenient time or transferred in stored form to a geographically separate system.

The difference between a quality music system and a pressure recording system is the frequency spectrum in which each operates. The audio (music) system has by far the broader frequency spectrum: from 30 Hz up to 20 or 30 kilohertz. At very low frequencies, though, a music system is unresponsive. This is as it should be, since one hears very little below 20 cycles (although one can *feel* organ pedal tones of 16 Hz). As for the pressure system, it does not perform much above the 100-cycle range, but does respond all the way down to 0 Hz or d.c. That is, it will indicate steady state pressures as well as low frequency changes in pressure.

As an historical aside, amplifiers able to cope with steady state signals were called d.c. amplifiers not because they could handle direct current, but because the interstages in the amplifier had a configuration known as direct coupling. Such amplifiers were subject to baseline drift, however. A second type of amplifier, providing baseline stability, employed capacitive coupling between the stages. Owing to the capacitive coupling, this species of amplifier could only process oscillatory signals or alternating currents. Such amplifiers could, however, be utilized for the recording of steady state phenomena if the incoming signal was repetitively interrupted or chopped, or caused to modulate (change the amplitude of) a higher frequency carrier. In this form the signal could pass through the capacitor-coupled amplifier. The envelope of the chopped signal constituted a faithful reproduction of the steady state phenomenon under observation.* Amplifiers of this type were called carrier amplifiers.

A resistance strain-gauge transducer will operate with either a carrier amplifier or a direct-coupled amplifier. A transducer of the differential transformer type, however, operates only with a carrier amplifier. Differential transformer transducers are now rarely used clinically.

Transducers

Transducer is the general term for a component that converts a mechanical force into an electrical signal or vice versa. Examples are phonograph pickups, microphones, and loudspeakers. In a pressure transducer slight displacement of a mechanical element causes a proportional change in the electrical signal emanating from the device. A very stiff diaphragm is attached to the displacement element so that changes in pressure applied to the diaphragm are faithfully translated into displacement and then to electrical signals. The principle is simple; but for the device to be linear over a wide range while retaining a modicum of ruggedness, intelligent design and exquisite care in fabrication are essential. These constraints contribute significantly to the high cost of pressure transducers.

---

*For further discussion see Geddes.[22]

The details of construction and operation of pressure transducers are adequately described in other texts.[22][77] In general terms displacement of a mechanical element in the transducer causes a directly proportional change in the electrical resistance of fine wires within the unit. The resistance wires are incorporated in a Wheatstone bridge, the characteristic of which is that a very large change in signal across the bridge occurs with only a very slight change in the resistance of any of its limbs. If the bridge is excited by a carefully controlled electrical source, then changes in output voltage will faithfully reproduce changes in pressure applied to the transducer diaphragm. The excitation voltage for the transducer is provided by a special circuit in the preamplifier.

Because the output signal of a transducer is a function of both pressure and excitation voltage, transducer specifications include a term that indicates a certain number of microvolts change in output signal per volt of excitation for every 10 mm Hg change in pressure. This is the sensitivity of the transducer. A typical nominal specification is 50 microvolts/volt of excitation/10 mm Hg pressure.

In the earlier days when pressure measurement was just evolving out of industry and the laboratory into a clinically useful tool, transducer sensitivity was determined by the design convenience of the several manufacturers. Even within a specific brand and model of transducer, variation in sensitivity was encountered from one unit to another. Therefore, ability to adjust the gain or amplification of the recording amplifier was mandatory if such transducers were to be useful. Statham, one of the dominant manufacturers, used a nominal sensitivity of 50 microvolts per volt per 10 mm Hg, and most production units were found to have sensitivities within plus or minus 5% of this value. Transducers standardized to within plus or minus 1% of the nominal sensitivity were available for a premium price. Transducers from other manufacturers, however, varied markedly from the nominal sensitivity elected by Statham.

During the middle 1970s there occurred a transition that received remarkably little verbal recognition, though it had significant effects on the type of equipment available to the clinician. Rather abruptly it became possible to dispense with some of the many controls that intimidated the uninitiated. First, a nominal sensitivity of 50 microvolts/volt/10 mm Hg seems to have been adopted as a standard sensitivity by all the major manufacturers. Second, production techniques became sufficiently refined that actual sensitivity of transducers adhered closely to nominal sensitivity without the need to specify or pay a special price for close tolerance. At the same time the virtually universal incorporation of solid state circuitry did away with the drift in amplification that had characterized some tube-type amplifiers. The net effect is that it is now possible to plug any of several brands of transducer into any of several brands of pressure amplifier with reasonable assurance that, if the system works at all, it is accurate to within 1%.*

The cables attached to transducers contain four extremely fine wires within a braided metal sheath or electrical shield. The cable is vulnerable to abuse by torsion and traction, particularly where the cable enters the base of the transducer and also at the connector. The falling of a transducer support, with the transducer still in it, can result in the cable literally being ripped out by its roots. Sharp kinking along the course of the cable will cause metal fatigue and eventually lead to breakage of the tiny conductors. When not in use, the cable should be stored in gentle loops, not tightly folded; and when the cable is extended, particular care should be exercised to insure that the loops are not converted into kinks. The cable should not be run over by other equipment nor stepped upon. Repair is costly and time-consuming and the outage of needed equipment is inconvenient.

THE PREAMPLIFIER

The preamplifier receives the small electrical signal from the transducer and performs initial amplification. It contains the controls necessary for zeroing and calibrating the incoming signal. The controls and their labels are so variable from manufacturer to manufacturer that the prudent operator will not fail to consult the instruction manual before attempting to operate the equipment.

Though a multiplicity of controls allows a preamplifier to be used with a broader choice of transducers characterized by different sensitivities and operating ranges, such versatility is irrelevant with respect to clinical blood pressure measurement. A transducer of 50

---

*There is no reason, save inertia on the part of both manufacturers and users, why all transducers and amplifiers cannot be fitted with a single type of compatible connector.

microvolt sensitivity suffices for observing the entire physiologic range of pressures, venous as well as arterial. A superfluity of controls only increases price and the complexity of operation. Equipment designed to operate only with transducers of 50 microvolt sensitivity, therefore, has few controls requiring user adjustment: a range selector and a zero setting.

Music amplifiers are expected to have a flat frequency response* over the entire audible spectrum. By the same token it would be expected that amplifiers utilized for pressure measurement would offer fidelity throughout the frequency spectrum of interest—from 0 to 50 Hz (or even to 200 Hz). Some amplifiers do, others do not. Some models roll off as low as 8 Hz. This means the amplitude response of the amplifier at 8 Hz will be only half that at 4 Hz, and pulsatile components of still higher frequency will simply not be perceived by the measurement system. Pulse tracings processed through such amplifiers will enjoy immunity from systolic overshoot or ringing introduced by a grossly underdamped hydraulic coupling system; but this agreeable smoothing of the signal is obtained at the price of throwing away high frequency data. Whether loss of data means loss of information is a debatable question to be examined later in this chapter. It suffices here to note that the enlightened investigator does not throw out or filter raw data in the absence of a conscious decision that the data are irrelevant. Few amplifiers are labelled on the front panel as to frequency response.

An output jack or tap is often provided at a point in the circuitry where the analog signal has been amplified to about plus or minus 2 volts. This allows for convenient capturing of the signal and its transfer to other recording or storage devices.

The Power Amplifier

From the preamplifier the signal is passed to the power amplifier where it acquires additional amplification to drive a readout device such as a galvanometer. The power amplifier may contain additional amplification controls or allow adjustments

---

*The relative amplitude of input to output signal is constant regardless of frequency.

peculiar to the readout mechanism, or it may have no external controls at all.

The Readout

It is at the readout that one encounters a wide range of options in merchandising features. With respect to medical equipment, the appearance of the equipment often seems more important to the prospective purchaser than what the equipment does and how effectively it performs.

The readout with the most venerable lineage is the *direct writer,* electronic successor to the smoked drum kymograph. Engineering improvements such as feedback and low mass pens have overcome the disadvantages of drag, inertia, and curvilinear scales that characterized earlier direct writers. (These handicaps have kept many serious investigators wedded to the photographic recorder despite the latter's messiness and the frustration of not being able to examine the tracing till it was developed.)

Ink jet pen recorders afford improved high frequency response relative to hot stylus recorders, and modern versions are said to be less delicate and incontinent than their forebears.

Nothing beats the electron for minimum mass and ease of control; so the *cathode ray tube* (CRT)—albeit something of an antique—continues to lead the pack with respect to immunity from display artifacts. It is also the least expensive analog display. Multiple traces, representing several channels of analog information, can be displayed on the face of a single cathode ray tube using high speed electronic switching. The process is called multiplexing or time multiplexing.

Unfortunately the familiar bouncing ball trace is ephemeral. How can it be engrossed? The addition of a Polaroid camera affords a permanent record of the CRT face. The camera finds wide use in the laboratory and in such clinical procedures as echo ranging, but is not generally useful in the operating room and intensive care unit. To secure a permanent record from a multiple-trace CRT, one manufacturer utilizes a fiberoptic light pipe to project a band of the CRT face onto a moving strip of sensitive paper that can be developed by intense ultraviolet light. The record is physically less than optimum; the cost, formidable.

An increasingly popular type of display utilizes a CRT with a single electron gun, just as in the bouncing ball display. The electron beam, however, does not simply undulate as a faithful mimic of the electrical signal amplified from the transducer. Instead, the scanning electron beam is controlled by sophisticated elements from computer science. The key element in this display system is the *shift register*.

The shift register is a memory device with locations to accommodate 1024 words in sequence. Each word is actually a number that represents the amplitude of a 4-millisecond segment of the electrical analog of the pressure pulse contour (or any other signal under observation). Since 1024 x 4 milliseconds = 4.096 seconds, the shift register can remember about 4 seconds worth of information.*

The word in each of the 1024 locations in the shift register is composed of 8 bits, a bit being an element representing either a logic state "0" or logic state "1." Since the numbers zero through 255 can be represented in the binary system by 8 bits, a word stands for any one of 256 discrete levels of amplitude. The required transformation from a continuously varying analog signal to a discrete number is performed by an electronic component aptly named an analog-to-digital converter or A-D converter.

Through a process to be described in a moment, words sequentially loaded into the first location of the shift register march on down the line—from one location to the next, only one word in each location—till the first word is lodged in the last (or 1024th) location in the register. Note that this word in the last location of the loaded shift register is actually the first word or oldest piece of information loaded into the register (by the write operation, also to be described shortly), while the *last* word is in the first location of the register and is the most recent piece of information (Figure 5-2).

Timing is the key to operation of the shift register and associated components. A master clock emits a pulse every 4

---

*The sampling rates, sweep speeds, and other specific numbers in this description are taken from data kindly provided by Hewlett-Packard Company, Medical Products Group, Waltham, Massachusetts 02154. Other manufacturers may use somewhat different values, but principles and orders of magnitude are similar. In this description, some numbers will be rounded to make them more manageable.

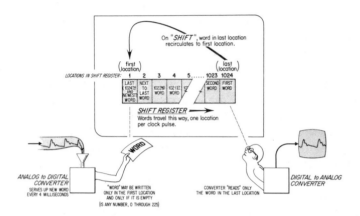

On "*SHIFT*", word in last location recirculates to first location.

LOCATIONS IN SHIFT REGISTER: 1 2 3 4 5 ..... 1023 1024

(first location) (last location)

| LAST 1024TH AND NEWEST WORD | NEXT TO LAST WORD | 1022ND WORD | 1021ST WORD | 10 | | SECOND WORD | FIRST WORD |

SHIFT REGISTER ⟶
Words travel this way, one location per clock pulse.

ANALOG to DIGITAL CONVERTER
SERVES UP NEW WORD EVERY 4 MILLISECONDS

"WORD" MAY BE WRITTEN ONLY IN THE FIRST LOCATION AND ONLY IF IT IS EMPTY
(IS ANY NUMBER, 0 THROUGH 225)

CONVERTER "READS" ONLY THE WORD IN THE LAST LOCATION

DIGITAL to ANALOG CONVERTER

Figure 5-2 Shift Register

microseconds (250 thousand pulses per second). There are other timing circuits that operate at different frequencies, but all are synchronized through the master clock. Of the secondary timers, one gives marching orders to the shift register.

Two commands to the shift register are allowed: (1) recirculate, or (2) write and recirculate.

If the order to recirculate is given, every pulse of the master clock causes each of the words in the register simultaneously to shift downstream a single notch to the next location. A shift occurs every 4 microseconds. The word that is shifted out of the last location in the register is recirculated directly into the first location. After 1024 pulses of the master clock all the words will be back in their original locations in the shift register; the shifting halts. Elapsed time: 4 milliseconds.

The recirculate operation simply recycles the words within the shift register. *Reading* of the words is accomplished through a digital-to-analog converter that applies to the vertical deflection plates of a cathode ray tube a voltage proportional to the numerical value of the word in the last location of the shift register. Only the word in the last location of the register can be read. Reading does not affect the word; it remains intact, to be recirculated into the first location upon the next pulse of the master clock.

The players and the basic rules of the game have been established. Next consider what happens if (1) the electron beam is caused to start a trace from the left edge of the cathode ray screen at precisely the moment the shift register is ordered to recirculate, (2) it takes the electron beam exactly 4 milliseconds to traverse the screen from left to right; and (3) during this traverse, the vertical displacement of the trace is made proportional to the numerical value of the word that is in the *last* location of the shift register at each 4-microsecond interval in real time. The result of this precision drill is that all the words in the shift register will be read individually in sequence and painted onto the screen as the point of light generated by the electron beam makes a sweep from left to right in 4 milliseconds. The oldest word—now back to analog form as a vertical distance—will lead off the display at the left edge of the screen, while the most recent word (the one that went into the shift register last) is represented by the electron spot as it reaches the right edge of the screen. In 4 milliseconds, then, the fact of the CRT is painted with an undulating line that is a facsimile of the 4 *seconds'* worth of information contained in the register memory.

After the left to right sweep of the screen is completed, there is a mandatory pause in the shift register activity. This pause allows the electron beam to move back to its starting point. (The beam is blanked so there is no trace of its swift return to the left edge of the screen.) Certain other operations also may take place during the mandatory pause. Recirculation, however, is not allowed; all the 1024 sequential words are frozen in their register locations. The pause duration is brief: just a few pulses of the high frequency clock, undiscernible to the viewer. Then a recirculate cycle can begin anew. So brief is the mandatory pause—perhaps 40 microseconds—that for practical purposes the synchronized operation to (1) recirculate, (2) read, and (3) sweep reoccurs every 4 milliseconds.

During each recirculate cycle any given word always fetches up at the last location after exactly the same number of clock pulses. This means that the particular word will be read onto the screen at exactly the same left to right locus that it had during the preceding sweep. The result is a bright trace that appears stationary on the screen. This is the freeze feature of the shift register display.

How is new information added? This is accomplished by giving the other timing command: *write* and recirculate. (Write refers to writing *into the memory,* not writing onto the CRT screen.) First, though, we must go back to the analog signal. As it comes from the amplifier, the analog signal is sampled 250 times a second: the stream of new data is chopped into pieces each 4 milliseconds long. The A-D converter looks at each piece, takes its average amplitude, and converts this into an 8-bit number (word) which is served up to the shift register. It is another rule of the game, though, that only the first location can accept a new work (and no shift register location can contain more than one word at a time). Therefore the shift register is unable to accept a new word unless the first location in the shift register is vacant. If the first location already contains a word, then the A-D converter simply throws its own word away and serves up a new one 4 milliseconds later.

It is the write part of the recirculate command that creates a vacancy in the first location, and time is crucial. The command to write/recirculate can be given only just before the end of the mandatory pause. On the command to write, the entire contents of the shift register are clocked ahead one notch. (All shifts require only 4 microseconds, and this is no exception.) But with the write command (as opposed to recirculate), the last location is forbidden to recirculate its word back to the first location. Instead, last location's word is thrown out and simply vanishes forever! (As per routine, last location receives a word from his next neighbor upstream.) Lo!, a vacancy now exists at the first location; whatever word has been readied by the A-D converter is now slipped into the first location on the same clock pulse without further orders. A recirculate cycle then begins with the very next 4-microsecond clock pulse. The CRT sweep is triggered also, and in the succeeding 4 milliseconds the whole memory is read and displayed. Remember that the shift register threw away the oldest word, worth 4 milliseconds in real time, so the trace commences with what used to be the *second* oldest word, and a new 4-millisecond piece of data now appears for the first time on the right edge of the screen at the tag end of the sweep.

Though a word is worth 4 milliseconds, any word is read and displayed in 4 *micro*seconds. On the present sweep, then, each word will strike the screen 4 *micro*seconds (real time) ahead of its locus on the preceding sweep. If the screen is 20 cm across and is swept from left to right in 4 milliseconds, this means each word will strike the screen 0.2 mm to the left of the position it held on the preceding sweep. Let the operation continue in this mode, with a new piece of data being written into the register at the end of each mandatory pause, followed immediately by recirculation, and the tracing will appear to march across the screen from right to left (at a rate of 50 millimeters per second on a 20 cm screen). Each new piece of data appears at the right side of the screen and disappears at the left side 4 seconds later. This is the moving trace display mode.

At the flick of a switch, the observer can change the command from write/recirculate to recirculate and the tracing will freeze to allow closer scrutiny.

Once the shift register, clocks, and logic components have been provided, variations of the display can be effected through relatively simple manipulations of the timing, blanking, and sweep circuits. The moving trace and the freeze have been described. Another variation is the erase bar display in which a vertical blank stripe moves from left to right across a motionless trace, the bar appearing to wipe out old and lay down new data in its wake.

The scanning electron spot, through other manipulations of its control mechanisms, can be put to a variety of time-shared tasks. For example, if two shift registers are provided, the contents of each may be displayed on alternate 4-millisecond sweeps of a CRT with a single electron gun. The zero level of the sweep is shifted downward on the screen an appropriate distance before the sweep for the second register has commenced, and after that sweep it is moved upward to start the next reading of the first register. When two shift registers are available, the contents of the first may be recirculated into the second, there to be frozen in display—at the touch of a button—while current data acquisition and display continue with the first register.

A single-gun CRT can readily display four, or even eight, shift register memories. Each register may process a separate channel of physiologic information or, as just indicated, the registers may be cascaded to provide as much as 32 seconds of continuous display of one incoming channel.*

A single package of electronics, containing the desired number of shift registers, can drive any number of CRT screens strategically

---

*This approaches improvidence as a means of storing data that are ultimately evanescent, and one must consider tape or paper as more appropriate for storage and retrieval of observations spanning more than a few seconds.

placed for visibility—an advantage in the coronary care unit setting, for example.

Alternating with its 4-millisecond sweeps to display a physiologic function, the electron beam may be given 4 milliseconds in which to perform quite different operations such as generating lines or bars denoting limits or rates.

It is not apparent to the casual observer that the CRT trace is being refreshed and the information updated as infrequently as every 32 milliseconds (as is the case in an 8-trace display). The *coup d'oeil* is carried off by ultilizing smoothing filters, by careful choice of phosphors coating the tube face, and by taking advantage of the persistence-of-vision phenomenon. The eye-cortex system does not discern flicker until images are renewed at something less than the home movie rate of 16 times per second, while each of 8 traces on one display can be updated and painted more than 30 times each second. Even though each shift register is itself updated every 4 milliseconds, it is well to remember that the visually pleasing display actually consists of 4-, 8-, 16-, or even 32-millisecond blocks of averaged data strung together and artificially smoothed by filtering. The digital origins of the apparent analog tracing are exposed in the display's readout of a slowly decaying pressure signal.*

Many of the real as well as cosmetic attractions of the shift register display have been enumerated in the course of describing its principles of operation. The prime limitation of the shift register display is cost: 4-second shift register memory adds nearly $1000 to the cost of a monitor.† A complete monitor package providing two channels of information including alarm limits for the ECG and a preamplifier for pressure measurement, but with conventional bouncing ball display, can be purchased for little more than the cost of two 4-second shift register memories alone (without amplifiers and CRT). While the freeze and other features of shift register methodology may have some merit in clinical settings where sporadic arrhythmias are likely and significant, there seems little justification for general use of shift register techniques to display

---

*Only the signal for CRT displays is digitized. The signal continues in analog form through the power amplifier and on to the strip chart recorder—if provided.

†True through 1977. Technology and the marketplace could effect change.

the ECG in operating rooms and surgical intensive care units; and there is no merit in thus displaying pressure contours.

The rate of sampling of the information fed into the A-D converter determines the faithfulness of the reconstructed wave form. Optimally, the sampling rate should be at least twice—and prefereably several times—that of the highest frequency in the original analog signal. Diagnostic electrocardiographic equipment is expected to have a flat frequency response up to 60 Hz, so a shift register sampling rate of 250 Hz would seem adequate.[60] Moreover, as a practical matter, a high frequency cutoff as low as 30 Hz does not materially degrade clinical electrocardiographic monitoring. By the same token, one would expect a sampling rate of 250 Hz to be more than adequate for clinical display of pressure phenomena. Yet, it is observed that the tracings presented by contemporary equipment are unduly smoothed, devoid of the high frequency elements that one is accustomed to seeing in conventional oscilloscope displays. (A possible explanation: with an 8-channel display, the effective sampling rate for any one channel is only 31 Hz, barely adequate to reproduce a 15 Hz wave component.)

Digital display. This popular mode fails to provide necessary information, and confers an aura of authenticity upon values that may be inaccurate if not irrelevant. Substantiation of this criticism follows.

Inspection of the pressure pulse contour as it is displayed on the oscilloscope not only affords information about the patient, but provides continuing ability to assess the *quality* of the observation process itself. New personnel rapidly acquire the ability to recognize good and poor quality tracings. The facility is more than academic: when using the pulmonary artery catheter, recognition of the damped or occluded tracing is essential in order to avoid distal lung infarction due to the catheter being in the wedge position. The observer who relies on digital display forfeits the indices of quality conveyed only in the pattern of the analog display.

As pointed out in Chapter 3 on the pressure pulse and its modifications, peak systolic pressure may be determined by either of two components in the pressure pulse. The two peaks tell different things about the heart and circulation; there may be 50 millimeters or more difference between the two, and neither may be absolutely valid owing to resonance in an underdamped hydraulic coupling system. None of these facts can be appreciated by the electronics of the digital display when it is set to read systolic pressure. The circuitry merely picks out the highest point on the curve and displays this number with witless authority.

Digital displays are useful when selecting a discrete value out of many, as when tuning a specific frequency on a radio received. However, a locus on a continuum is more logically represented in scalar format and is better perceived in this mode of display.

Despite their cost (about $300 each) and inappropriateness, digital displays continue among the options most frequently selected by purchasers of new medical equipment.

OPERATION OF PRESSURE MONITORS

The various knobs, terminology, and procedural details are so inconstant from manufacturer to manufacturer that resort should be made to the instruction book appropriate for a particular device. Ready availability of an instruction manual, along with condensed operating instructions attached to the device, are hallmarks of a quality organization.

Calibration

Zero setting preceds calibration. Formerly complex and tedious, zero setting is now quickly accomplished (with the system open to air) by adjustment of a single control on most modern monitors.

Pressure recording systems are calibrated in two ways: (1) electronically, and (2) by application of pressure. Pressure calibration in turn comes in two varieties: (a) static, and (b) hydrodynamic.

Electronic calibration is really a dodge, an artifice—not true calibration. This is how it works: ulitizing a mercury manometer, a specific pressure is applied to a new transducer. The gain (amplification) of the recording system is then adjusted so the recorder shows the true manometric pressure. The transducer is then opened to air.

In the next step, the output voltage of the transducer (still open to air) is changed a specific amount by connecting a calibrated precision resister into the circuitry. Note is then made of the pressure reading of the recorder. This number becomes the calibration number or gauge number (the terminology varies) for that particular transducer. The transducer is appropriately tagged; better still, the gauge number and the model of the corresponding preamplifier are engraved on the transducer.

Whenever that particular transducer is used, the same precision resistor (or one of identical value) is inserted into the amplifier circuit, and the gain of the amplifier is adjusted so the recorder indicates the calibration number previously determined. The resistor is then removed from the circuit and the system is ready to record.

With some brands of monitors (Electronics for Medicine, for example) the precision resistor is incorporated in the circuitry of the preamplifier. In another brand (Lexington), the precision resistor is physically contained in the transducer's connecting plug. In either case, a switch on the amplifier places the precision resistor in or out of the circuit.

Electronic calibration is merely a gross indication that the system may be working. It is not necessarily an indication of the accuracy, and certainly not of the linearity, of the transducer and its connections. Indeed, in some rack-mounted instruments such as the Hewlett-Packard line, the electrical signal for calibration is injected between the preamplifier and the power amplifier. On moving the calibration lever the machine will display the right pressure even if a transducer is not connected to the preamplifier!

What *is* the zero reference level? If the transducer was air-filled for calibration and for zero setting, then the plane of the transducer diaphragm is the zero reference level. If zero was set with fluid in the transducer, then baseline level is the horizontal elevation of the air-fluid interface at that time (whether it be an open port on a stopcock on the transducer or the end of the fluid column in connecting tubing open to air).

Static calibration. The serious clinician insists on calibration by pressure. He will see to it that his systems are calibrated against mercury at the beginning of each series of observations (and against a column of saline for low pressure measurements) and periodically rechecked during the course of the exercise.

For calibration purposes it does not matter whether the system is filled with air or liquid. A mercury manometer is connected to the transducer and, through a T-connector to a hand bulb or large syringe, pressure is applied to the transducer. Four or more readings should be taken over the range of anticipated extremes of pressure to insure linearity. (Transducers may be damaged by heavy thumb pressure on the diaphragm, for example, and become nonlinear. It has been our experience, though, that if the transducer works at all, it is likely to remain linear.)

Hysteresis is commonly observed. That is, pressures displayed in stepwise upward pressurization of the transducer are slightly but distinctly different from those observed during stepwise depressurization.

As noted in the section on transducers, a growing number of transducer-pressure monitor combinations need no gain or amplitude adjustment, and therefore have no control for that purpose. The Cal button provided is merely a system function test device and is no guarantor of accuracy.

Lack of immediate access to a mercury manometer and fittings should not discourage one from performing a pressure check if there is the least anxiety or insecurity about the pressure readings. Michael Snider of the Massachusetts General Hospital has pointed out that one is never far from a column of saline that can be quickly and easily applied to the transducer to produce a known hydrostatic pressure. One simply removes the flush solution bottle from the intravenous tubing that connects it to the transducer, and turns the stopcock so the transducer diaphragm is "looking at" the fluid column. The drip chamber is then held so that the meniscus above an unbroken column of fluid is 68.0 cm above the zero reference level. This column of saline is equivalent to 50 mm of mercury.

Although 68.0 cm is longer than most CVP (central venous pressure) measuring scales, one may fabricate sticks or chains of appropriate length. A handy utensil may turn out to be just the right length: as shown in the illustration (Figure 5-3), one brand of CVP catheter is packaged in a tube that is just 1 cm (or one fingerbreadth) short of the water equivalent of 50 mm of mercury.

If one becomes vague about the relationship between centimeters of water and millimeters of mercury, the dual calibration of the airway pressure dial on many anesthesia machines serves as a handy reference.

The matter of *dynamic calibration* will be discussed later in this chapter in the section on Design Considerations.

Flushing

If the connecting system were filled with air, only mean pressures would be obtained; if the system were allowed to fill with

118

blood, it would clot. The purpose of flushing, therefore, is to keep the system free of both air and blood.

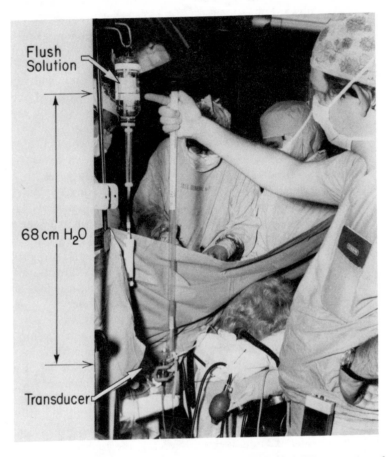

Figure 5-3 Quick static check of transducer calibration against column of water (saline) is demonstrated by Michael Snider Ph.D., M.D., under field conditions.

In a minor variation on the technique described in the text, the drip chamber is filled (to provide an unbroken column of liquid) and the height of the flush solution bottle is adjusted so its fluid level is 68 cm above the zero reference line. The stopcock is then turned to connect the transducer to the flush solution line rather than to the patient. Monitor should read 50 mm Hg. Package for CVP catheter happens to be almost 68 cm long, providing handy measuring stick.

Whether a continuous slow flush or intermittent flushing is employed is a matter of user preference. Many who spend their days in the operating arena favor the intermittent flush system. When this system is utilized, respect must be entertained for the possibility of embolism (discussed shortly under Hazards). The continuous flush devices do not provide for adequate initial debubbling of the hydraulic system.*

As to the choice of flushing medium, arguments may be offered for saline alone: first, glucose-containing flush solutions provide an excellent carbon fuel source for contaminant organisms.[73] Second, plastic, nonwettable surfaces do not promote clot formation. A protein-covered surface, however, stimulates clot formation; this process is not significantly inhibited by dilute heparin. In the absence of electrolyte, proteins are reluctant to remain in solution. Thus, an electroyte-free flushing solution will tend to favor deposition of plasma proteins on the otherwise nonwettable surfaces of indwelling catheters and cannulas, resulting in acceleration of clot formation despite heparin. An appropriate flushing solution, therefore, is one that contains at least a small amount of electrolyte.†

Although electrical conductivity of a solution is enhanced by the presence of electrolyte, from the practical viewpoint there is no real compromise of electrical safety when salt-containing flushing solutions are used.

Other possible hazards related to flushing systems are delineated in following subsections.

Infection

Invasive pressure monitoring constitutes yet another breach of the ill patient's armor against infection. This breach should not be taken lightly. However, the care afforded cannula entry sites is

---

*Preliminary studies show a loss in frequency response when a continuous flush technique is used.[3]

†Though the value of heparin in arterial flush solutions has not been evaluated, to the best of my knowledge, heparin (1,000 U/L) has been shown to prolong the viability of chronic venous infusion routes (by retarding onset of phlebitis).[15]

observed to be highly ritualistic and not uncommonly leads to disruption or pulling out of vital lines. In the ordering of priorities, security comes first lest the patient risk exsanguination or be unnecessarily subjected to yet another puncture, or to time-consuming probing to find vessels that may already have been much abused.

Pressure-sensing devices in dialysis equipment and in intensive care units have been implicated in the transmission of bacterial and viral infection from patient to patient.[73][33] Associated monitoring procedures have also caused infection by nosocomial organisms.* While bacterial contamination of equipment should be readily controllable, there is no evidence that any of the cold sterilization techniques (including ethylene oxide) have any effect on the serum-carried viruses associated with hepatitis. The long and futile search for a transducer which can be autoclaved should perhaps be abandoned in favor of disposable dome-diaphragm units introduced in the mid-1970s.

Disposable dome-diaphragms may affect transducer sensitivity, and the manner of application of the disposable unit substantially affects frequency response of a transducer directly coupled to a test chamber.[19] These findings may not be clinically relevant inasmuch as the prime factor influencing frequency response is the connecting tubing between patient and transducer. There are no frequency response data on tubing and transducers, in combination, employing disposable dome-diaphragms.

A worthwhile custom is the daily changing of all solutions, tubing, and fluid paths down to the disconnect site closest to the patient.

Electrical Safety

When electricity is passed from one extremity to the other, a current of about 100 milliamperes is required to initiate ventricular fibrillation. This is the amount of current drawn by a 12-watt light bulb at 120 volts. If current is led directly to a small contact on cardiac tissue, however, then ventricular fibrillation might be initiated by currents as small as 100 microamperes.

---

*See also the discussion of hazards relating to the pulmonary artery catheter, Chapter 6.

The higher figure applies if a cannula in a peripheral artery were to serve as a port of entry for electric current. Even though the contact is subcutaneous, current fans out from the contact point and largely fills the volume of the conductor offered to it. It is simply not true that blood vessels lead electricity to the heart "just like a wire." The low current values capable of initiating ventricular fibrillation apply only when there is direct cardiac contact. A terminal floating free in a cardiac chamber requires much larger amounts of current to produce an effect, just as a pacemaker wire in poor contact cannot predictably initiate pacemaking.[55]

Electricity cannot ooze out of a single contact. Current only flows when there is a complete circuit; and electrocution can occur only when the victim becomes the component that closes a circuit in which a lethal current can flow. In order for a hazardous situation to exist, it must be possible to find a way for electricity to get from a voltage source, travel through the pressure monitoring equipment and connections, through the individual, and then through some other route back to the voltage source. In practice this is not easy to do, despite fanciful hypothetical proposals. Indeed, if one uses plastic connectors and stopcocks, the only metallic element in the liquid column to the patient's body is the transducer diaphragm. Even in those older transducers that were not advertised as isolated, this diaphragm (and the transducer case) are not connected to any electrical element nor to the ground shield in the cable. Indeed, the transducer will not operate properly if there is an element short to the case. The prudent may wish to mount older transducers in insulated holders or use disposable dome-diaphragms, but there is no justification for premature discarding of perfectly serviceable equipment.

The threat of electrical injury has been inflated wholly beyond reason, while the complexities of achieving electrical safety in the hospital have been both confused and grossly exaggerated. These things have come about partly through ignorance, but largely have been contrived in order to maintain a favorable merchandising climate that spuriously forces obsolescence of older equipment. The fundamentals of electrical safety are quite simple, and should be assimilated by those regularly using electrical equipment, whether in a hospital or at home.[10]

Other Complications

The voluminous literature on vascular injury allegedly associated with arterial cannulation at the wrist in adults is out of proportion to the relatively few misadventures associated with extensive use of this valuable technique. Loss of digits or significant tissue is virtually unknown except in association with protracted low flow states which ultimately claim the patient's life.

The true incidence of severe vascular compromise is not known, but is estimated to be 0.01% of all cannulations on the basis of 10 years' close clinical observation at the Massachusetts General Hospital. During this experience Allen's test was not performed regularly, either because the patient could not cooperate or the test was considered unpredictive. Furthermore, many patients are known to have had ipsilateral sequential invasion of the ulnar artery as well as the radial. Statistical data on the imprudence of this practice will never become available owing to poor recording and the fact that it flies in the face of recommendations pontificated out of hindsight.

In the severely burned adult we have not shied from utilizing the femoral artery when necessary, and have encountered no complications. This is not to say that they will not eventually be encountered. However, forebodings expressed by our colleagues in vascular surgery are not supported by relevant experience with long-term invasion of the femoral artery for angiographically-directed control of hemorrhage utilizing vasopressin infusion.

Though departures from conservative practice are not to be taken lightly, those dealing with the very sick must cope daily with diminishing alternatives in caring for patients critically ill for long periods of time. The clinician's burden is not eased by those declaming from podiums far removed from the battlefield.

A bulky dressing should not be placed over the cannulated extremity, even in children. The digits should be continuously exposed to the watchful glance of all who pass.

Regarding composition, surface finish, and configuration of cannulas as related to tissue acceptability, the literature is unsatisfactory. Tapered cannulas have been condemned, yet the tapered portion of the condemned cannula lies outside the skin, not in the artery! With respect to preferred material, variations in formulation and fabrication, and particularly the surface characteristics of the cannula, have more effect on tissue compatibility than the basic polymer (such as vinyl, propylene, or Teflon).[59]

Disconnection of components is a common, major, and preventable complication. Medical personnel seem unaware of a characteristic of plastics: by their very nature they have poor dimensional stability. Plastics tend to creep.* All plastic stopcocks and Luer fittings can, after a little time, always be tightened just a little more. When a cannula is successfully inserted, it should be carefully dried. Then the cannula and adapter should be seized with coarse, dry cloth, dry rubber gloves, or clean dry hands, and forcefully fitted together. The security of the cannula must be such that it can pass the Laver test,† that is, it must be possible to suspend the cannulated limb by the connecting tubing without avulsing the cannula. Free ends and projecting caps that can catch on bedclothes are to be avoided.

In a perhaps understandable quest for security, some personnel regularly restrain the patient's arm in a posture of marked hyperextension. Not only does this posture soon become painful, but it may result in motor weakness of long duration.

Lowenstein et al. have shown that exuberant flushing of the wrist cannula may result in retrograde flow into the carotid.[43] Cerebral embolization of air or clot is conceivable if caution is not exercised.

Arteries and arterioles are unwilling receptors of irritant and vasoactive substances. Intraarterial injection of drugs intended for intravenous infusion may be disastrous.

DESIGN, PERFORMANCE, AND TESTING OF PRESSURE MONITORING SYSTEMS

Of necessity this section begins with an essay on the operation of the marketplace with respect to clinical monitoring equipment. Appreciation of the facts of mercantile life is prerequisite to appreciation of why we have certain types of equipment, and why

---

*Polycarbonate (Lexan) is least likely to show this property.
†M.B. Laver, M.D., Massachusetts General Hospital.

that equipment may seem to perform in ways that are often less than satisfactory. The problem is not simply one of engineering: we clinicians are a large part of the problem.

After a frankly editorial preamble, I will tender some proposals on specific design and performance considerations, including tentative solutions to what will remain unsolved problems until there is more general perception of their very existence. These unsolved—and perhaps unsolvable—problems relate to modification of the pressure pulse by the hydraulic coupling system. This will be another look, therefore, at considerations initially presented in Chapter 3. Finally, I shall review the methodology of calibrating performance of clinical monitoring systems.

Monitors, Science, Commerce, and Regulation

What is a pressure monitoring system supposed to do? How should it perform? The questions are appropriate and straightforward, but the answers are difficult. The difficulty lies in the fact that the questions are not recognized as ones that ought to be posed! Perception of the need to ask is one of the best kept secrets in the practice of acute care medicine.

Ordinarily astute and skeptical physicians set aside the methodology of the scientist when dealing with monitoring equipment. This syndrome is all the more paradoxical inasmuch as the measurement problems discussed in this text are known to investigators in the laboratory, and have long been delineated in available literature. The roots of this paradox stem in part from the clinician's naive regard for hospital equipment, coupled with his arrogant disdain for instruction manuals. The clinician expects his equipment to work and to give the right result immediately on its installation without further effort on his part.

Such behavior is in marked contrast to procedures and expectations in all other scientific disciplines. Pertinent is Lenfant's caveat: "...Any researcher spends considerable time learning about and checking the instruments that he is going to use; this is, in fact, the first requirement of research apprenticeship. Each physician, no matter how busy he might be, must assure that he or anyone else responsible to him will learn about his equipment. It is fallacious to believe that a fool-proof instrument...can be developed..."[41]*

While an unqualified definition of the right pressure monitoring system is not possible at this time, I shall attempt at least to define the boundaries of pertinent concerns by analyzing four questions:

1. What does he (the clinican) *need?*
2. What does he *want?*
3. What can he *have?*
4. What does the customer *buy?*

The fourth and last question, interfacing at the marketplace, is the easiest to answer: customers buy features and packaging, not performance. There is nothing new in the engineering of pressure measurement. Contemporary devices provide no information that was not available through older, simpler, less costly devices. Only the packaging is new—and packaging sells the product.

Who buys this product? The purchaser is rarely the individual destined to cope with a monitoring system day and night in the operating room or care unit. Nor is the customer the person who ultimately pays for the system. The patient pays.

Who *does* buy equipment? How are purchase decisions made?

The mechanics and methodology of hospital purchasing are long overdue for ruthless ventilation. With one exception, the few studies available do not merit citation either as to content or literacy. The exception is the extraordinary report by McNeil and Minihan that perceptively analyzes the contemporary compulsion to develop defensive strategies in medical practice owing to rising performance norms being enforced upon the hospital sector. These authors describe the genesis of defensive strategies in three stages.[48] There first occur crises, real or otherwise, that arise from breakdowns in more sophisticated device technology. The second stage sees proliferation of standards and norm-defining agents putatively generating solutions to problems (which may be more

---

*Even the nonprofessional aircraft pilot must demonstrate knowledge of the prescribed accuracy and tolerance of navigation instruments in order to pass his examination for licensure. Before utilizing the instruments in flight, he must verify that their accuracy has been checked within a prescribed period, and that there is a written record of the findings.

imaginary than real). The third stage is exuberant foliation of norm-enforcement channels. Significantly, though, the norm-enforcers are isolated from the norm-definers! In an attempt to cope with harassing, threatening, and sometimes irrational intrusions by norm-enforcers, the hospital develops defensive strategies that affect "the decision-making criteria which hospital administrators use, either consciously or unconsciously...." The results may not be salubrious. As McNeil and Minihan put it: "Given the dreadfully complex and fragmented regulatory environment, administrators may constantly buy ever more exotic technology to protect themselves from the vulnerabilities of the existing technology. This is a shell game that only works, however, as long as funding sources can continue to afford the sky-rocketing costs of often unworkable technology."[48]

Not only do hospitals generate defensive strategies to cope with identifiable norm-enforcers, but open season has been declared on the medical establishment by litigious bounty hunters and opportunistic professional crusaders. Defensive strategies, provoked by bureaucratic harassment spiced with the fear of legal entanglement, constitute a "plausible explanation of the widespread adoption [by hospitals of a particularly expensive but unnecessary electrical system]."[48] "Even if these devices don't prevent [an alleged danger], the hospital in any liability suit could claim that it had bought the 'latest' in technology to control equipment failures."

The answer to Who buys? is *hospitals:* they issue the purchase orders.

Not only are defensive strategies involved in equipment acquisition, but the elegant appearance and putative power of acquired systems are also hospital and departmental status symbols, much like icons or totems arrayed on the tribal turf. The successful manufacturer designs for this untutored market; and save for the longer distance between the pockets of the vendor and the payor (a consideration that further favors extravagance), the medical equipment market is driven by much the same instincts that maintain the thriving market for automobiles loaded with extras having little to do with basic transportation. This is not to say that the manufacturer is at fault. He can, and will, make anything the customer will buy; and to stay in business, the manufacturer must satisfy prevailing market demands.

Should there be any doubt that unessential features sell medical devices, visit the plant! The final assembly benches are crowded with monitors festooned with intricate alarms and featuring solid state, computerized innards. From the faces of these designer-styled boxes, stacks of digital readouts redundantly proclaim information already displayed on the adjacent, prodigiously expensive, bright screen oscilloscope. These overdesigned, overengineered creations are about to be dispatched to the same hospitals that daily beseech public help in balancing their budgets.

The fourth question, then, was easy to answer: it is ordinarily *not* the user who actually purchases equipment. Purchase decisions are predicated on how the equipment looks, what it is said to offer, or what it is believed to offer. Equipment thus obtained may not provide appropriate solutions to clinical needs.

Now, as to what can the clinician *have,* and what does he *want?* Because these third and second questions are intertwined, the conscientious manufacturer finds himself on the horns of a dilemma. Insofar as electronics are concerned, the manufacturer can build anything the clinician might want. The problem is that the clinician commonly doesn't know what he wants! Unable to offer conceptualization of his needs, he merely *reacts* with annoyance when confronted with a system that fails to behave in accordance with his visceral expectations.

Thus, it is only when the product reaches the field that the manufacturer learns whether or not he has satisfied the needs of the user. If the manufacturer has failed and feels constrained to make amends, he has recourse only to the process of trial and error in an effort to satisfy his field service people and preserve the reputation of the company. Even if there exist lines of communication between user and manufacturer, the former is of little help because he literally doesn't know enough to define what is wrong.

This sanguine view of clinical monitoring is neither fictionalized nor academic. The prevailing situation is costly, mutually frustrating, and not just a little ridiculous—as the following case history indicates:

A major manufacturer of monitoring equipment distributed a clinical unit that was very well received. Owing to manufacturing exigencies, it became necessary to modify the amplifier circuitry in a later production run. As the newer units were put into service, company representatives started calling in from all over the country to convey their customers' bewilderment and dissatisfaction with the newer product. The monitors, it was claimed, gave systolic pressure readings that were outrageously high. Upon investigation, it was found that the original manufacturing run of monitors had a sharp rolloff quite inadvertently built in at 12 Hz. The amplifier acted as a low pass filter, and it was unresponsive to frequencies above 12 Hz. In designing the circuit for the newer production run, however, a different engineer had simply done that which seemed electronically feasible and appropriate; his effort led to production of an amplifier that easily handled frequencies up to 50 Hz. The customers who bought these higher fidelity amplifiers were (in their view) plagued by pressure recordings that looked less smooth and gave systolic pressures that did not correspond to the assumed "real pressure" as determined by other methods. (It was the excessively high numbers displayed by digital readouts that caused particular annoyance.) The manufacturer redesigned the unit, restoring the frequency limit to its previous low level of about 12 Hz. This third production run has been well-received.

Finally, what does the clinician *need?* First, he needs a system that will provide information useful in the management of his own patients. Second, systems should allow meaningful comparisons between data obtained by different observers at other times and places.* This brings us to a discussion of monitor performance.

How Should a Pressure Monitoring System Perform?

The performance question is unanswerable at this time. Theoretically, the optimum system should have a flat frequency response throughout the range of interest. Flat frequency response means that, for an input signal of constant intensity, a graph of the system output plotted against frequency will be a smooth horizontal line. Put another way, the relative amplitude of the input and output signals will be constant over a specified frequency range.

---

*It could be argued that only this second constraint mandates actual calibration of the performance characteristics of a measurement system. The situation is somewhat analogous to the amateur musician, playing alone, who may find enjoyment while fingering just a few notes on an instrument in tune only with itself. But to play his part in an endeavor by a group of professionals, the musician must command the full range of his instrument and assure that it is tuned to concert pitch.

The general principle for obtaining a flat frequency response is to design the system with a resonant frequency well beyond the highest frequency encountered in any signal to be observed. Two problems arise in attempting to apply this general principle to pressure monitoring systems: first, the upper limit of the range of pertinent frequencies in the pressure pulse has not been defined. Just as in the earlier days of electrocardiographic investigation there was no standard for system frequency range, so there is no current standard for performance of direct blood pressure recording systems. Indeed, no common interest group is even considering the question!

While experienced investigators suggest that the upper limit of pertinent frequencies in the pressure pulse spectrum may be as low as 12 or 15 Hz, the fact is that the issue of upper limits has not been systematically studied in the context of acute care environments of the 1970s wherein gross manipulations of contractility, peripheral resistance, and other hydrodynamic variables are commonplace.* It has been reasoned that an upper frequency limit of five times the pulse rate would suffice to include all relevant data; but the pulse rate is merely the repetition rate of an event and should not be confused with the frequency content within the event envelope. The disregard of data beyond frequencies as low as 6 to 10 Hz would appear cavalier. Perhaps useful information about inotropic phenomena may be contained in frequencies as high as 20 or even 50 Hz.?

The second problem resides in the fact that a pressure measuring system is composed of two *subsystems:* (a) an electronic system, and (b) a hydraulic system. While there is no problem in obtaining a pressure monitor that has a flat frequency response from zero to 100 or even 200 Hz as far as transducer and electronics are concerned, the hydraulic connecting system to the patient is quite another matter: within the 10 to 20 Hz bracket fall the resonant frequencies of the highly underdamped hydraulic systems employed to join peripheral arterial cannulas to strain gauges. Since there is no immediately foreseeable way of recording pressure components in

---

*Clinical equipment at the Mayo Clinic, 1977, incorporates a 15 Hz filter with rolloff in excess of 40 db per octave. McDonald in 1960, quoted by Strandness and Sumner, suggests that acceptable amplitude distortion tolerance is 5% at 15 to 20 Hz.[68]

that frequency range without their being subject to considerable amplitude distortion, we find ourselves in a box. What this means in terms of debasing clinical data, and what to do about it, are discussed next.

Performance Specifications: Realities and an Interim Proposal

Though the secret has been carefully kept from clinicians, it has long been known to engineering and laboratory people that characteristics inherent in the hydraulic connecting system markedly affect the quality of the displayed pressure pulse and the amplitude of its components. On the presumption that nothing but noise is contained in frequencies above approximately 15 Hz, commercial as well as in-house monitors have been manufactured with filters that sharply attenuate frequencies above this range. Granted that this artifice produces pressure pulse tracings that may be more socially acceptable, the wisdom of the operation is questionable. How can it be established whether data do or do not contain information if the data are thrown away before being examined?

Electronic filtering may make up for deficiencies of the hydraulic coupling system; but this is makeup in the cosmetic sense, not a cure for underlying blemishes. The results of filtering are not only that data of possible value have been discarded without evaluation, but also that serious traps have been set for the unwary clinician—he who presumes to serious investigation but is unaware that the data presented by the monitor have been electronically rigged.

The traps already contain victims, for some monitors are filtered; other brands are not; virtually none is labelled! While diastolic pressures are not affected, the filtered type of monitor will simply not "see" extremes of systolic pressure displayed by an unfiltered system. This means that different conclusions may be drawn regarding such essential matters as pressure modification by drugs and the comparison of different treatment modalities, simply owing to the signatures of the recording systems. Furthermore, arithmetically determined mean pressures between filtered vis-á-vis unfiltered systems are not comparable, and this in turn invalidates comparison of derived values for peripheral vascular resistance.

It should be clear that the attempt to draw precise quantitative conclusions about *flow* on the basis of the contour of the pressure curve is all the more a fool's enterprise if one does not even surmise the presence or absence of filtering.

Interim suggestions. Until the necessary work is performed that will delineate the information value of specific frequencies in the peripheral pressure pulse, what should be done about the present anarchic situation?* Enlightenment is always a good place to start. It is suggested that electronic filtering is probably not a bad idea; but the presence or absence of filtering should be a user option, and the degree of filtering must be indicated by a label that is conspicuous as well as specific. The moronic "diagnostic" vs "monitor" labeling of some electrocardiographic monitors is to be avoided. Rather, a specific frequency should be cited at which filtering begins, along with an indication of the slope of attenuation. *Only with institution of specific numbers* will it begin to be possible to compare values obtained from differing monitoring systems. It will also be necessary to quantitate the characteristics of the hydraulic coupling system utilized. How to do this will be described later in this chapter.

Since the problem of fidelity lies in the connecting tubing, why not do something about the tubing? Omitting it altogether raises the resonant frequency to 40 Hz or more, even with the use of a relatively large-displacement transducer. However, omitting the tubing is simply not practical in the clinical setting. A reasonably flushed system incorporating a 4-foot length of tubing can be expected to have a resonant frequency of 20 Hz or better—but it is grossly underdamped. Why not build into the tubing an appropriate resistance so that damping can be improved with but little concurrent reduction of resonant frequency?[39] Tubing manufacturers were approached with the idea years ago, but none has taken it seriously.

A procedure *not* to be recommended is placing an air bubble in the system (even in the transducer where it will not inadvertently be flushed into the patient). While an air bubble produces a pressure pulse tracing that is cosmetically pleasing, the transformation is accomplished at an unacceptable cost in frequency response: the resonant frequency drops from 20 Hz to 5.5 Hz—and with only a slight increase in damping factor!†

---

*Happily, the current situation is more damaging to the credibility of investigators than to the lives of patients.
†Personal observations.

Consideration of *phase shift* has been postponed to this point because it would have been awkward to discuss in parallel with frequency response. Phase shift is really of little concern in the clinical pressure monitoring situation owing to the futility of attempting to draw profound conclusions about timing of centrally occurring events on the basis of observations at the distant periphery. Inconstant and unanalyzable phase shifts in pressure pulse components have occurred by the time the pressure pulse even reaches the interface between patient and monitoring system. Suffice it to say that phase lag increases linearly with signal frequency in an optimally damped* system, making corrections for phase shift possible. To avoid any significant phase shift at all, though, requires that the resonant frequency of the observation system be 10 or more times that of the highest frequency in the processed signal.

Putting Together a Pressure Monitoring System

Yet to be written is the treatise that satisfactorily sets forth the optimum plan for a pressure measuring system that is convenient and practical for use in the operating room or at the acute care bedside, and will also be of service in clinical investigation. Some general statements are warranted, however, based on analogies with other types ofelectromechanical systems such as those for the reproduction of music or voice.

First, there is no point in overengineering the system beyond the user's needs or comprehension. If only spoken voice is to be reproduced by a sound system, for example, then phase shift is of little consequence, and there is no need to engineer high frequency capability perceivable only by the family dog. One can end up amplifying noise at the expense of intelligibility, with both frustration and erroneous conclusions as results.

Second, the quality of the system should be appropriate to the quality of the signal source—the data processed. Symphonic fidelity is not required of a sound system if the program input is limited to scratchy records and music to chew gum by. In observation of the pressure pulse it is dubiously appropriate to provide a digital

---

*Defined in Chapter 1.

readout that displays—to three significant figures—a value that may have undergone 50% or more distortion in amplitude.

Third, the quality of the components should be relatively uniform throughout the system. It is improvidence, indeed, to spend thousands of dollars on a high-frequency ink jet recording galvanometer when the assembly of components includes a preamplifier that rolls off at 8 Hz.

While it is important to know the accuracy of a system, accuracy is not the top priority. In ascending order, priorities are (a) accuracy, (b) reliability, and (c) repeatability.*

In summary, the major problem in pressure monitoring systems lies in the hydraulics and not in the electronics. Blotting out potentially informative data, owing to unwitting utilization of electronic filtering, is not the way of the wise. Meaningful comparison of data acquired through different systems and at different times requires calibration and documentation of the dynamic performance characteristics of entire systems. How to do this will be examined in the next section.

Hydrodynamic Performance Testing of Systems

In the process of recording a pressure pulse, input frequencies above the system's resonant frequency will be blotted out, while signal frequencies in the neighborhood of the resonant frequency undergo amplification if the system is underdamped. It is appropriate, then, to have some appreciation of the resonant frequency and the damping of the system one employs.

Two methods are available for overall quantitative evaluation of a pressure monitoring system (cannula, connecting tubing, and stopcocks—along with transducer and electronics). The methods are:

1. Step function or square-wave tests
2. Sweep-frequency test

The two methods are similar in that an input signal of known composition is applied to the system. The output of the excited

---

*Herrick, quoting Spencer regarding analogous concerns with vascular flowmeters.[32]

system is evaluated as to faithfulness in replicating the input signal. The methods differ with respect to the character of the test signal and in the complexity and expense of the equipment required to perform the test.

The square-wave technique is artless, but shows readily the degree of ringing (lack of damping) and resonant frequency. Square-wave testing is crude but to the point: rather like slamming an automobile door and listening for rattles.*

For square-wave testing an abrupt change in pressure is applied to the system: the signal at the input is "stepped" from one steady state to another. Subjected to this stress, the system will oscillate momentarily and then settle down at the new steady state value. The frequency of the observed oscillation indicates the resonant frequency of the system. The exuberance of oscillation provides a measure of the system's damping.† It is technically difficult to create a virtually instantaneous increase in pressure at a system input, but a sudden *drop* in pressure can provide equivalent information.

To perform the test the fluid-filled system is connected to a small chamber that may be conveniently pressurized by air from a hand bulb. The precise pressure is of no consequence; 100 mm of mercury will suffice. The top of the test chamber is formed by a tightly stretched rubber diaphragm. After pressurization of the system the chart recorder is run at high speed, and the diaphragm of the test chamber is ruptured by a pointed blade or a hot needle held in a soldering iron. The diaphragm must actually explode so there is instantaneous release of pressure (otherwise, spurious damping is introduced). The resonant frequency of the oscillating system is determined from the wave periods on the recorder, while damping may be calculated or derived from available tables.[20] (See Figure 1-2 for test example.)

The advantage of this system is that it requires but a simple test chamber, fabricated for only a few dollars. Some scientists disparage the notion that significant information can be derived from a technique so naive as literally striking a system and observing how it vibrates.[47] However, since most of the world's great music has

---

*Square waves were introduced in Chapter 1.
†Hansen attributes use of the technique to Frank shortly after the turn of the century![31]

been composed on instruments tuned in precisely this manner, the technique is hardly devoid of some merit. This simple test quickly and ruthlessly provides unflattering evidence regarding the fidelity of one's pressure observation activities. Observed values range from 10 to 25 Hz for resonant frequency, with damping consistently as low as 0.2. It is humbling to be confronted with evidence that the display on a kilo-dollar monitor is largely conditioned by a few dollars' worth of disposable plastic tubing or a gratuitous air bubble.

The other method, the sweep-frequency test, requires equipment costing hundreds of dollars. In this technique, a sine wave signal from an electronic frequency generator is passed through a high quality, high power audio amplifier.[13 67 47] The amplifier drives a current-to-displacement transducer fabricated from a loudspeaker driver or a galvanometer motor. The transducer becomes a pressure generator when rigidly connected to a diaphragm that forms part of the wall of an otherwise rigid test chamber. A reference transducer is set in another part of the wall of the chamber. The assembly is completed by providing ports for attachment or insertion of test cannulas and connectors. The compressible volume is kept small and recesses that might trap bubbles are avoided.* Elegant craftsmanship is required in the fabrication of this device—of which few examples exist. Most are homemade, though a commercial model is available.†

The test chamber serves to generate a sinusoidal pressure of constant amplitude over a span of frequencies provided by the electronic frequency generator.‡ As the frequency generator is swept

---

*Yanof et al. in a classic article describing an exquisitely fabricated piston device, review the intricate concerns pertinent to accurate generation of sinusoidal pressures.[76]

†Millar Instruments, P.O. Box 18227, Houston, Texas 77023

‡Long familiar with the tenuous low frequency response of sound transducers, I harbor visceral uneasiness about the unqualified accuracy of this method. Use of feedback to provide flat frequency response from the pressure generator is discussed by Brodhag.[9] (As an aside on the wisdom of deriving sophisticated parameters from low fidelity recording techniques, Brodhog offers the trenchant comment: "The diagnostic value of a dp/dt measurement in a system that has a 12 db peak at 22 Hz is rather questionable.")

from very low to progressively higher frequencies, the amplitude of the output signal is continuously recorded. A typical tracing on a strip-chart recorder, therefore, appears as a ribbon of ever increasing density as the frequency is swept from low to high. The sides of the ribbon are parallel, indicating constant amplitude output. At some point, however, the ribbon widens, peaking of the response occurring at the system's resonant frequency. The response to still higher frequencies is rapidly attenuated. The amplitude distortion at resonance is a measure of the system's damping.

If it is agreed that a system response within 5% of the true value is a reasonable target, and the system is underdamped (0.2 or less), then only those signals with frequencies at or below one-fifth of the resonant frequency of the system will be recorded with accuracy.[76] Thus, utilizing an underdamped system with a resonant frequency of 15 Hz, only those phenomena with frequency components of three per second or less can be recorded without exuberant amplitude magnification. Since early systolic components of the pressure pulse embrace frequencies of 8 or 10 Hz and upward, the implications with respect to fidelity of clinical blood pressure monitoring are humbling.

CONCLUSION

That the technique is invasive and the requisite devices formidable, bestows on direct blood pressure measurement an aura of authenticity that is not warranted owing to the vagaries inherent in the methodology and equipment. Systolic values, in particular, are likely to be a function of the way the values are obtained. Derived parameters and indices are similarly suspect.

It is suggested that scientific journals publishing clinical studies relating blood pressure values and derived indices require that investigators specify the performance characteristics of the measuring system utilized.

6 Low Pressure Measurement

THE EQUIPMENT

The same transducers and electronic equipment utilized for direct measurement of arterial pressure serve also for low pressure measurements. It is necessary only to increase the gain (amplification) of the preamplifier by a factor of about five. An attenuator knob or range switch is provided for this purpose.

An increase in gain means there will be increases in the amplitude of noise, artifact, and error—along with the signal.

For strip-chart recorders using conventional ECG paper with 1 mm squares, it is convenient to let each major block of five squares equal 25 mm Hg pressure for the arterial tracing, and 5 mm Hg pressure for low pressure recording. Analogous layout of the scales on the oscilloscope face will provide approximately full scale deflection of 0 to 200 mm Hg for high pressure and 0 to 40 mm Hg for low pressure observation.

Leveling of low pressure transducers is critical. While a few centimeters of vertical elevation or depression of an arterial transducer matter little, such discrepancy may profoundly affect conclusions drawn from observations of low pressure such as the pulmonary capillary wedge pressure.

137

Electronic calibration can be misleading when utilized on low pressure systems inasmuch as small errors in the calibration signal—trivial on the arterial pressure scale—are multiplied when the amplifier gain is increased for low pressure observation. If one intends to take the absolute numbers seriously (rather than just observe trends in the low pressure modality), then it is prudent to check the calibration of the system against a column of saline. Remember, also, that mercury is about ten times heavier than water—but "about" is imprecise, and a 40% error will be introduced if the correct conversion factor is not used.*

THE PULMONARY ARTERY CATHETER AND HOW IT WORKS

The Swan-Ganz Catheter

Use of a flow-directed balloon-tipped catheter† to gain access to the pulmonary artery in man was described in 1970 by Swan, Ganz, Forrester, Marcus, Diamond, and Chonette, who credited the principle to the work of Lategola and Rahn in the early 1950s.[69] General availability of reliable catheters with appropriate performance characteristics is owed to manufacturing expertise acquired in refinement of the Fogarty embolectomy catheter, of which the Swan-Ganz catheter is a lineal descendent.

Coincidental with commercial availability of the balloon-tipped catheter, ripening of factors both economic and technical rendered feasible the application of another long-known principle: thermodilution for determination of cardiac output.

Inserted by the Seldinger technique, the flow-directed catheter with thermodilution capability is one of the most exciting medical advances of the 1970s. Into the hands of the clinician has been placed a tool for diagnosis and continuing evaluation of therapy that formerly was restricted to an elite of initiates in the recondite temples of the cardiac catheterization laboratory. With relative ease, and as often as necessary with no added risk to the patient, it is now possible to nail down two of the three variables in the critical

---

*The correct conversion is 1 mm Hg = 1.36 cm water.
†N.L. Pace has provided a recent comprehensive review.[52]

equation that relates pressure, flow, and resistance, and from which are derived the values for work and power.

Though graced with this valuable tool, we must exercise caution in drawing conclusions from clinical observations inasmuch as simple d.c. circuit computations are not wholly applicable when dealing with pusatile energy and the hydraulic power transferred from ventricles to the periphery. In the systemic circulation, fortunately, the pulsatile component about the mean (or d.c.) is only 10% to 20% of the total power.[12][68] Therefore, calculations based on mean values may not be too wide of the mark. In the pulmonary circulation, however, this is not the case; for compliance is high, resistance low, and the pulsatile component of power is a much larger fraction of the total and is highly dependent on heart rate.[68][49]

The inflatable balloon on the Swan-Ganz catheter serves three purposes. First, just as a toy balloon wafted on a breeze is followed by its tethering string, the balloon on the catheter rides in the blood stream and directs the catheter into and through the right heart and into the pulmonary artery and one of its branches. Fluoroscopy is not required. Second, the balloon is carefully fabricated so that, when inflated, it almost envelops the stiff tip of the catheter. The latter is thus prevented from impinging upon cardiac structures susceptible to mechanical excitation. Third, the balloon easily wedges into an arterial branch, isolating the catheter orifice from the pulmonary arterial pulse. The tip "sees" only the distal or downstream pressure that is a close and faithful approximation of left ventricular filling pressure.

Before the advent of the balloon-tipped catheter, it had been necessary to insinuate a tiny catheter tightly into a small pulmonary artery branch, insuring that catheter and vessel were perfectly concentric to achieve complete obliteration of flow past the catheter but yet not obstructing its orifice. Tedious to execute, requiring fluoroscopy, a successful wedge reading was considered indicative of pressure in the pulmonary capillaries. Thus the expression pulmonary capillary wedge pressure (PCWP or PCW).* Figure 6-1 is a representation of why a wedge pressure indicates left ventricular diastolic pressure. The principle is really quite simple: there is no

---

*Of dubious legitimacy is the acronym PAWP, for "pulmonary artery wedge pressure, since the wedge is a *venous* pressure.

pressure differential across a resistance if there is no flow. Considered another way: the pulmonary vessels downstream from the locus of a wedge are simply a prolongation of the catheter itself.* Theory and method are supported by simultaneous measurements confirming identity of directly and indirectly measured left atrial pressures.[40]

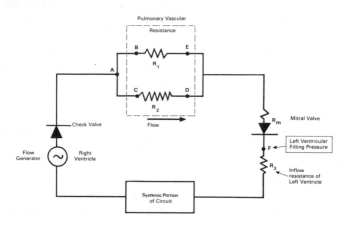

Figure 6-1a Pressure Relationships in the Pulmonary Circuit 1. A catheter floating in pulmonary artery branch A-C "sees" pressure at C. Pressure C is same as that at A and at B.
2. D,E, and F are all connected to each other, so pressure at these points is the same. (Resistance across mitral valve is assumed to be negligible.)
3. But A is *not* equal to pressure at F owing to flow across the pulmonary vascular resistance (PVR). Pressure difference is equal to product of flow (cardiac output) times pulmonary vascular resistance.
(a) Pressure at F cannot be inferred since its determinants are unknown.
(b) It *can* be inferred, however, that mean pressure at F is always some value less than mean pressure at C. (Blood does not run uphill.)
4. In most instances pressure at F is only slightly less than pressure at A because pulmonary vascular resistance is very low. Pressure drop across the lung remains small even with large values of cardiac output. (This is not the case if PVR is abnormal.)

---

*(1) Pulmonary arterioles do not intercommunicate at the precapillary level. (2) The caliber and compliance of a catheter are irrelevant to observation of steady state pressure or the mean of pulsatile pressure. (3) Inasmuch as bronchial arterioles do anastomose with pulmonary arterioles just proximal to the pulmonary capillaries, it is not clear why a moiety of systemic arterial pressure is not sensed when the PA catheter is wedged.[14] The

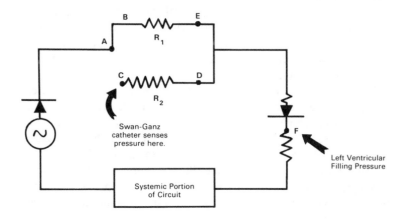

Figure 6-1b Catheter in Wedge Position Let a balloon-tipped catheter occlude the pulmonary artery branch at C, and let catheter orifice look downstream. Now pressure "seen" at C is same as that at D—and also at E and F.

Proof: If there is no flow across R_2 (route blocked by balloon), there will be no pressure drop across R_2. Therefore, C = D which is also equal to ventricular inflow pressure at F (again ignoring mitral valve resistance). This is true no matter how high the PVR, and regardless of cardiac output.

It has been suggested that (1) the vertical location within the lung of the catheter tip may condition the values observed for pulmonary artery pressure, and (2) that position may similarly affect PCW readings in that the numbers observed may reflect airway rather than vascular pressure.[4] While the first proposition is difficult to accept at all, evidence for the second has been offered by Roy and his colleagues who present a lucid and perceptive explanation for the observed phenomena.[58]

---

bronchial arterial supply must represent a very high resistance source in a circuit closed by a very low resistance load (represented by the pulmonary vessels downstream in the wedged segment). Some of the difficulty in obtaining a satisfactory wedge after the catheter has been in place for a considerable period may relate to dilatation of broncho-pulmonary arteriolar anastomoses.

Attainment of the wedge position is indicated by disappearance of the dynamic appearing pulmonary arterial tracing and replacement by the more sedate wedge tracing.

Why is the wedge tracing not pulsatile inasmuch as the catheter is looking downstream into the left atrium, certainly a generator of pulsatile flow? There are at least two reasons for the relatively non-pulsatile appearance of the wedge signal. First, little change in *pressure* is generated within the atrium owing to the very low impedance offered by the normal mitral valve and by the left ventricle in diastole. Second, any retrograde pressure pulse generated passes initially into the highly capacitant pulmonary veins and then into the resistance presented by the pulmonary capillaries. This configuration, a parallel capacitor followed by a series resistance, is the classic design for a smoothing or a ripple filter to change a pulsatile signal into a steady one. Thus, only highly damped vestiges of the atrial pressure wave—of small amplitude to begin with—are discerned in the wedge tracing.

V waves are large-amplitude excursions, time-delayed relative to ventricular systole, superimposed on the pulmonary artery tracing and the PCW tracing. The official explanation for V waves is "functional mitral valve incompetence." (A more likely origin of V waves is discussed later in this chapter.) Though the official explanation of their genesis may be fictional, the dynamic qualities of V waves are of practical value in determining whether, in the presence of an exuberant V wave and associated artifacts, the catheter is really in the wedge position or is still looking at the PA (pulmonary artery) pressure.

The criteria for determining whether balloon inflation and deflation accomplishes wedging and unwedging are: (1) quality change, (2) phase change, and (3) mean change. The first two criteria are more conveniently appreciated if the PA and peripheral arterial traces are superimposed on the oscilloscope screen. Superimposition occurs automatically if the scales suggested earlier are used with a common baseline, since the peripheral arterial and pulmonary arterial pulses begin almost simultaneously, and each has a similar, sharply oblique upstroke.

As to *quality:* the V wave differs from the pulmonary artery pressure pulse in that the V wave is more smoothly rounded, its upstroke less steep, and the obliquity of the upstroke is similar to the downstroke. The V wave, then, is symmetrical, while an undamped PA pressure pulse is steep-fronted.

A less subjective discriminator is change in *phase:* as noted above, the PA and peripheral pressure upstrokes begin almost simultaneously. A V wave, however, is delayed in time relative to the peripheral (or PA) pressure pulse. Thus, if the wedge position has been achieved, there should be a readily discernible interval between the start of the peripheral pressure upstroke and the start of a V wave.

A final check is accomplished by comparing *means.* The mean PA pressure must be higher than the mean wedge pressure—however pulsatile—otherwise blood would flow from left atrium to right ventricle, a condition not associated with longevity. This check is accomplished by allowing the chart paper to run while the amplifier is swtiched to mean. After the stylus stabilizes, and with the paper still running (10 mm per second will do), the balloon is deflated. If a wedge had in fact been achieved, now a significant upward step in the stylus tracing should occur indicating that the amplifier is seeing something different, i.e., the PA pressure, and is computing its mean. If there is no step of 2 to 5 mm Hg or more, then suspicion should be entertained that a wedge had not been attained in the first place.

The terminal step in the exercise is to switch the amplifier back to phasic display and observe restoration of an undamped PA tracing, insuring that the catheter is not floating into a permanent wedge position. After recording a few beats, the chart paper is returned to slow speed for observation of trends. An entire sequence of observations, which engrosses mean values for later computations, can easily be performed in 30 seconds by an unassisted operator using but 10 or 12 inches of recorder paper.*

---

*I am indebted to Michael Snider, Ph.D., M.D. for introducing me to this efficient protocol.

Problems Peculiar to the Intracorporeal Catheter

There are two species of problems peculiar to using the Swan-Ganz catheter. These are (1) reading the pressure traces, and (2) reliably wedging the catheter. These problems arise because the catheter is continually subjected to two types of perturbation: (1) that due to its traversing the chamber of a contractile ventricle, and (2) agitation of the delicate plastic catheter free-floating in a pulsatile stream.

The catheter forms an almost complete loop in passing through the right ventricle. This loop is tightened and released with each contraction of the heart. The coiling and uncoiling of the catheter imparts axial acceleration to the fluid column within. This acceleration is sensed as pressure by the transducer. The result, blithely labeled catheter whip, is the inscription of spikes of noise upon the pulmonary artery pressure tracing usually just prior to, and at the end of, the systolic component. The whip artifact is analogous to the disturbance produced when one flicks a finger against the connecting tubing of an arterial pressure setup.

The spurious pressure signals, though of considerable amplitude, are of such short duration that mean pressure is not significantly affected; but the artifacts bedevil attempts to develop simple electronic methods of assigning numbers to PA systolic and diastolic pressures. Most monitors with digital displays are not particularly smart and will call out diastolic pressure as the lowest point in a series of values—artifacts or not. (This can lead to the physiologically improbable situation in which the PA diastolic pressure is much lower than the wedge pressure even in the absence of large V waves.) The experienced eyeball does a much better job of picking out peak and diastolic pressures amidst a series of artifacts.*

---

*Though it is deplorably unscientific to insert an uncalibrated air bubble into the transducer as a means of blotting out unwanted noise, perhaps there is an argument here for simple electronic filtering. A high-frequency filter of known characteristics would at least permit more confident comparison of data developed by different investigators. It is questionable whether accurate knowledge of the PA diastolic pressure is of sufficient importance to merit determination through sophisticated and expensive data processing techniques.

Consider now the end of the catheter floating in the pulmonary artery: it is not quiescent. Were we to enjoy the privilege of seeing the Swan-Ganz catheter regularly under fluoroscopy, we would be reminded that it is in constant motion. Even under normal conditions there is hilar dance: the pulmonary vascular blood volume changes with each beat. The aggregate capacity of the pulmonary vessels also waxes and wanes over longer periods of time in response to respiration, shifts of volume from pulmonary to systemic circulation, and as a reflection of changes in total blood volume. Thus, the catheter is subject to constant to-and-fro movement axially as well as laterally, while the entire apparatus is tending to be propelled outward toward the periphery of the lung and attain the wedge position even without inflation of the balloon.

The problem accrues still another dimension owing to the dynamics of inflation of the balloon. The catheter does not reside within a smooth-walled tube of fixed cross section. Rather, the artery is constantly expanding and contracting; and perforating its wall—like so many holes in a Swiss cheese—are the orifices of branches. Into any one of these holes may fall, or be obliquely extruded, the balloon in the process of inflation. Shin et al. have shown that the balloon *does* inflate eccentrically and may assume a variety of surprising deformations.[62]*

In view of the foregoing constellation of influences, it is no surprise that there will be problems over relatively short spans of time with both the pulmonary artery pressure measurement and wedge measurement. Far greater vigilance and experimentation are necessary in the management of the pulmonary artery catheter than in the case of a peripheral arterial measurement system, and a repertoire of methodology must be invoked for success. Slow inflation of the balloon may sometimes be best, while—another time—rapid inflation may achieve a wedge. A forceful flush with a few ml from a syringe may propel the catheter tip away from the wall of the artery or out of a persistent wedge position. Slight pulling back of the catheter is a common requirement after it has been in place for a number of hours.

---

*On inflating the balloon, the recording needle may jump to a high level instead of dropping toward a wedge pressure. One explanation is that the orifice at the catheter tip is pressed against the vessel wall except at the moment of peak systolic pressure so that the recorded pressure is clamped at a spuriously high level.

Flushing

Selection of the flushing medium (saline vs dextrose) is dependent upon considerations already reviewed in the section on Operation of Pressure Monitors in Chapter 5.

While commercially available continuous flushing mechanisms are a convenience, these will not suffice for initial debubbling of the system. Removal of bubbles sequestered in the interstices of transducers and stopcocks requires vigorous and repeated flushing. This is best accomplished by forceful flushing with a syringe at the transducer end of the system, and a vigorous aspiration of fluid and trapped bubbles into a syringe at the patient end of the connecting tubing. The process may be repeated, after a pause, during the setup process.

A good pulmonary artery trace has a characteristic signature. I am reluctant to see filtering introduced into pulmonary arterial pressure measurement systems because the quality of the PA trace—its raggedness—is a criterion of the "goodness" of the recording: freedom from clots, bubbles, or impingement on a vessel wall.

Hazards

Hazards of the Swan-Ganz catheter include those related to its insertion. Carotid puncture occurs even in the hands of the most experienced. The event is not catastrophic, but is of concern in the patient about to be heparinized. Pneumothorax, hemothorax, and hemomediastinum are recognized complications of attempted entry into large vessels about the thorax.

Tangling of two foreign objects within the heart has been reported, and the presence of a pacemaker wire may be an indication for reversion to insertion and withdrawal of the catheter under fluoroscopic observation.

General considerations and putative concerns regarding electrical safety were presented in Chapter 5. Irritability observed in passage of the catheter through the heart is owed to mechanical stimulation.

When the presence of a thermodilution catheter is combined with use of the electrosurgical instrument (ESU), an awareness of observations in animals by Geddes and his colleagues may be in order: both irritability and endocardial burns were encountered when the ESU was used in experiments with intracavitary pacing wires.[23] Inasmuch as electrical insulation is relatively ineffective at high frequencies, there is a possibility (albeit far-fetched) that the thermistor probe or its wire might serve as a return path for part of the high frequency current during activation of the ESU.

When the ESU is employed in surgery on highly instrumented patients, I insist that a dispersive electrode with a large surface area be in contact with the patient.[1][34] It may also be prudent to disconnect the thermistor catheter from the cardiac output apparatus during activation of the ESU.

A rare but diastrous event is perforation of the pulmonary artery 6 to 36 hours after catheter insertion.

More likely to occur, but less catastrophic, is infarction of a distal lung segment owing to outward migration and permanent wedging of the catheter tip.*

Constant phasic display of the pressure signal is indicated, and observers should be able to determine that the pressure wave form originates from the pulmonary artery and is not a wedge tracing with a prominent V wave.

Right-sided septic as well aseptic endocarditis has occurred in association with venous pressure catheters and pacemaker wires. The Swan-Ganz catheter has been associated with thrombotic endocardial vegetation formation in the right side of the heart, but no association was established between the use (or nonuse) of the PA catheter and left-sided endocarditis.[27]

Flavobacterium harbored in an ICU ice machine has been linked to an outbreak of nosocomial bacteremia.† Appropriate concern should be afforded management of the ice bath and syringes for thermodilution procedures.

Infection and care of equipment are discussed also in Chapter 5. A great mystique (having to do with ointments, dressings, and

---

*It may be that what we call infarction is, in reality, pulmonary hemorrhage and not infarct. For a provocative—if not wholly satisfying—discussion of embolism, hemorrhage, and pulmonary infarction, see Dalen et al.[14]
†Stamm et al.[66] Myriad post hoc rituals proposed in this otherwise informative report are about as sensible as cooling of syringes prior to arterial sampling for blood gas determination—an unnecessary ritual that created the reported problem!

148

violations) has evolved which will not be treated here. Suffice it to say that contamination at the site of catheter entry is not the same as infection,* and that the consultant who recommends wholesale withdrawal of vital invasive lines should be prepared to replace them himself.

About Those V Waves

V waves observed via the Swan-Ganz catheter are popularly attributed to regurgitant flow from the left ventricle, the retrograde pressure wave being smoothed and time-delayed owing to filtering through the pulmonary veins and capillaries. The problem with this seemingly plausible explanation is that it does not fit the facts. When pressures are observed simultaneously via a pulmonary artery catheter and a left atrial catheter, the V waves are virtually identical in shape, amplitude, and timing at both sites (Figure 6-2). This would not be the case if the waves were created by regurgitant flow across the mitral valve.

An acceptable explanation for the V wave must describe a phenomenon that either evolves so slowly that there is no phase shift (time delay) in pressure rise between the left atrium and the pulmonary capillaries; or the pressure generating event must globally affect every part of the pulmonary venous outflow tract (including the left atrium) simultaneously in the course of each pulse cycle.

An explanation of the genesis of the V wave which satisfies the latter of the foregoing constraints can be structured on consideration of (1) flow characteristics in the pulmonary veins, and (2) the volume storage and volume dumping functions of the left atrium. The hypothesis to be presented eschews retrograde flow, pointing instead to periodic excess of inflow over outflow in the pulmonary veins and left atrium, these being conduits of generous but finite capacity.

---

*For review of contamination vs infection, references to local treatment of insertion sites, culture methods, and literature citations regarding intravenous catheters, see Maki et al.[44]

The origin of V waves. Clues to the formation of V waves are found in tracings of the *progressive* evolution and devolution of V waves following onset and cessation of nodal rhythm, Figures 6-2 and 6-3.

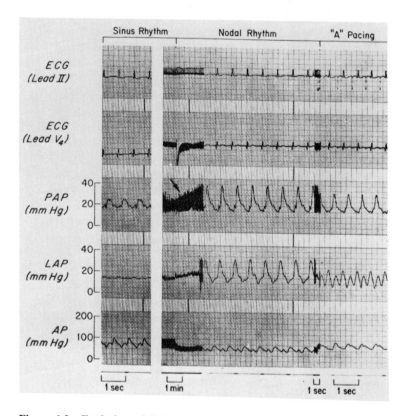

Figure 6-2 Evolution of V Waves Development of V waves occurs but gradually after transition from sinus to nodal rhythm (arrow, PAP strip). The V waves observed on the pulmonary artery tracing (PAP) are almost identical in phase with those observed directly from the left atrium (LAP). Institution of atrial pacing diminishes but does not abolish V waves. The LAP channel appears to have been recording mean pressure until just before onset of higher speed tracing. Deformation of arterial pressure tracing (AP) is due to intraaortic balloon pump. (Reproduced with permission of the publisher, from: Lappas, Demetrios G. et al. Cardiac dysfunction in the perioperative period. *Anesthesiology.* 47:117-37, August, 1977. New York: J.B. Lippincott Co.)

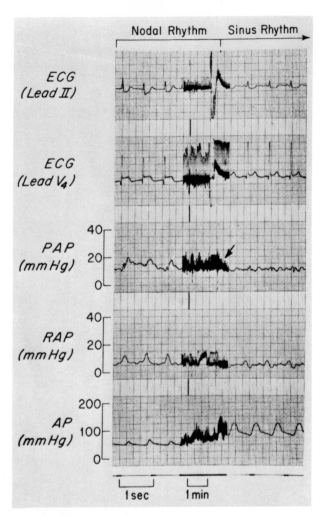

Figure 6-3 Devolution of V Waves V waves are prominent in pulmonary artery catheter tracing (PAP) during nodal rhythm. Electrical conversion to sinus rhythm is associated with *gradual* decline in amplitude of V waves in PAP tracing (arrow). The balloon catheter appears to have been wedged throughout this strip.

Disappearance of V waves from right atrial tracing (RAP) is somewhat more abrupt. Doctor Lappas reminds me that CVP and RAP tracings tend to lose their pulsatile quality when mean venous pressure is below 10 mm Hg. (Reproduced with permission of the publisher, from: Lappas, Demetrios G. et al. Cardiac dysfunction in the perioperative period. *Anesthesiology.* 47:117–37, August, 1977. New York: J.B. Lippincott Co.)

While flow into the capacitant pulmonary artery is highly pulsatile, flow into the pulmonary veins downstream from the pulmonary capillary resistance is somewhat more continuous. The left side of the heart thus is offered a fairly constant input. The left ventricle, however, can accept volume only periodically—when the ventricle is in diastole and the mitral valve is open. During part of each cardiac cycle, then, right heart output would pile up in the pulmonary venous system were it not for the left atrium. The normal atrium serves to store accumulating volume, then dump it into the relaxing left ventricle at precisely the right moment. Because the (pulmonary) venous-atrial system is highly compliant, normally no pressure changes occur even though volume changes are significant.

When the atrium is nonfunctional, as in nodal rhythm, the accumulate-dumping function of the left atrium is compromised. At the start of nodal rhythm the low pressure in the veins (and nonfunctioning atrium) may not be sufficient to translocate into the left ventricle a full stroke volume during the brief window of acceptance by the ventricle (particularly if the latter is stiff or less than normally receptive). As a result, volume progressively accumulates in the pulmonary veins. For an interlude of several beats, right heart output actually exceeds flow into the left ventricle. Since systemic vascular resistance hasn't changed, and left ventricle filling has decreased, a sharp drop in systemic arterial pressure may occur. Eventually the volume rise in the pulmonary veins progresses to the point at which capacity to dilate further without increased wall tension is reached. Now each left ventricular systole will be followed by a pulsatile pressure elevation in the pulmonary veins and left atrium, not because of regurgitant flow, but merely because flow across the pulmonary capillaries into the veins and atrium late in systole cannot exit till the left ventricle is next in diastole.

One would predict that the contour of a pressure pulse so generated would not be sharply inflected as from a regurgitant squirt; rather, it would tend to be smooth-contoured and symmetrical, resembling a cosine-squared pulse.* Moreover, the wave would be delayed in time relative to onset of pulmonary and systemic arterial systole. Such, indeed, is the appearance of the V wave.

When atrial function is restored, the V waves do not instantly disappear; rather, they gradually decline in amplitude over the course of several succeeding beats (Figure 6-3).

---

*Cosine-squared pulse is described by Gabe.[20]

These observations are consistent with the hypothesis that V waves may be encountered whenever the ordinarily flaccid pulmonary venous system becomes turgid and is obligated to operate on the steeply sloping part of its compliance curve.

VENOUS PRESSURE

> All animals are equal but some animals are more equal than others.
>
> George Orwell: *The Animal Farm.*

The steam has gone out of the 1950s romance with central venous pressure, though some still regard the procedure with tempered affection. It is true that trends and changes in venous pressure may be of significance even though the absolute value may not be wholly informative.

Since the procedure is one of those that often is not worth doing at all, it is probably not necessary to do it well. Therefore, reference will be made to two mythologies that serve unduly to distract and often waste time of acute care personnel. These mythologies are: (1) that some pressures are more central than others, and (2) that a transduced pressure is somehow more accurate than a saline manometric pressure.

Anyone who has tried to thread a catheter from the external jugular vein into the thorax knows that the process is not easy owing to valves, and particularly because of tortuosities and angulations in the vein at the base of the neck behind the clavicle. Owing to these same impediments the external jugular veins may be distended even though the central venous pressure is quite low. Once access to the internal jugular has been gained, however, there are no valves upstream from the tricuspid. Pressure is the same, regardless of flow, throughout any system that is free of valves and resistances.

It is not true, therefore, that a catheter tip must be within the thorax—the more "in" the better—in order to register a true CVP (central venous pressure). The only exception might obtain if the CVP is markedly below atmospheric; in that case, the vein might collapse, allowing the recorded pressure to equal that of the atmosphere.

Further evidence of the nonapplicability of this oft cited myth may be observed with the insertion and withdrawal of the

Swan-Ganz catheter via the neck: once the catheter is within the introducer, the same pressure is registered throughout the catheter's traverse to the tricuspid valve.

As to the second myth: is the venous pressure different when measured by a column of saline as opposed to a transducer? Obviously the fluid manometer has a much longer time constant than a transducer of small volume displacement; that is, it takes a longer time for the fluid to drain in or out of the manometer and thus come to a stable reading. This means that the liquid manometer displays time-averaged mean pressure. Could it also be that the hydraulics of the fluid manometer somehow "clamp" the observed pressure at a spuriously high value?

The hypothesis of nonequality was tested in two ways in the clinical setting. First, the CVP catheter was connected alternately to (a) a transducer via a 4-foot connecting line, or (b) a fluid manometer system, via a stopcock on the central venous pressure line. In a second series of observations, the CVP catheter was led to a transducer via a 4-foot connecting line, and the other port on the same transducer was connected to a saline-filled manometer. In this second series, the various stopcocks were so oriented that the fluid column was in continuity from the patient, through the transducer, and into the fluid manometer.

Before the venous pressure measurements were made, the zero level and amplification of the transducer recording system were calibrated directly against the fluid manometer utilized in the same series of observations. To secure a concordance within a few millimeters of mercury was the most difficult part of the whole operation.

At no time, either with the alternating or the in-line technique, was there a significant discrepancy between the transduced and the fluid manometer mean venous pressure readings.

There is no difference, then, between fluid manometer and "transduced" venous pressure readings provided (1) the transducer is meticulously calibrated and zeroed against the fluid manometer, and (2) the appropriate saline-mercury conversion factor for pressure is employed.

REFERENCES

1. Aronow, S. and Bruner, J.M.R. Electrosurgery. (Editorial) *Anesthesiology.* 42:525-26, 1975.

2. Bagshaw, R.J. Assessment of cerebrovascular hydraulic input impedance. *IEEE Transactions on Biomedical Engineering BME.* 23:412-16, 1976.

3. Bauld, T.J., Grant, R., and MacKenzie, D. Frequency response characteristics of blood pressure monitoring systems for ICU use abstracted. Presented at 12th Annual Meeting of Association for Advancement of Medical Instrumentation. San Francisco. 1977.

4. Benumof, J.L. et al. Where pulmonary arterial catheters go: Intrathoracic distribution. *Anesthesiology* 46:336-38, 1977.

5. Bertrand, C.A. and Pascarelli, E.F. Arm and leg blood pressures (letter to editor). *JAMA.* 227:942, 1974.

6. *The Bible,* King James version. Ezekiel, chap 1, verse 16.

7. Braunwald, E. Determinants and assessment of cardiac function. *N Engl J Med.* 296:86-9, 1977.

8. Brecher, G.A. and Galletti, P.M. Functional anatomy of cardiac pumping. Edited by W.F. Hamilton and P. Dow. In *Handbook of Physiology, Section 2, Circulation.* Vol. II, pp. 759-98. American Physiological Society. Baltimore: The Williams and Wilkins Co., 1963.

9. Brodhag, J.A. *Dynamic characterization of blood pressure measuring systems.* Pasadena: Bell and Howell Company, January 13, 1975.

10. Bruner, J.M.R. Fundamental concepts in electrical safety. Edited by S.G. Hershey. In *Refresher Courses in Anesthesiology.* Vol. II. Philadelphia: J.B. Lippincott Co., 1974.

11. Caldini, P., Permutt, S., Waddell, J.A., and Riley, R.L. Effect of epinephrine on pressure, flow, and volume relationships in the systemic circulation of dogs. *Circ Res.* 34:606-23, 1974.

12. Cox, R.H. Determinants of systemic hydraulic power in unanesthetized dogs. *Am J Physiol.* 226:579-87, 1974.

13. Crul, J.F. Measurement of arterial pressure. *Acta Anesthesiol Scand.* 11(suppl):135-69, 1962.

14. Dalen, J.E., Haffajee, C.I., Alpert, J.S. et al. Pulmonary embolism, pulmonary hemorrhage and pulmonary infarction. *N Engl J Med.* 25:1431-35, 1977.

156

15. Daniell, H.W. Heparin in the prevention of infusion phlebitis. A double-blind controlled study. *JAMA* 226:1317–21, 1973.

16. Elsner, R., Franklin, D.L., VanCitters, R.L., and Kenney, D.W. Cardiovascular defense against asphyxia. *Science.* 153:941–49, 1966.

17. Felix, W.R., Hochberg, H.M., George, M.E.D. et al. Ultrasound measurement of arm and leg blood pressures. *JAMA* 226:1096–99, 1973.

18. Flacke, W. and Alpher, M.H. Actions of halothane and norepinephrine in the isolated mammalian heart. *Anesthesiology.* 23:793–801, 1962.

19. Fox, F., Morrow, D.H., Kacher, E.J., and Gilleland, T.H. Laboratory evaluation of pressure transducer domes containing a diaphragm. *Anesth Analg.* 57:67–76, 1978.

20. Gabe, I.T. Pressure measurement in experimental physiology. Edited by D.H. Bergel. In *Cardiovascular Fluid Dynamics.* Vol. I, pp. 11–50. New York: Academic Press, Inc., 1972.

21. Geddes, L.A. *The Direct and Indirect Measurement of Blood Pressure.* Chicago: Year Book Publishers, 1970.

22. Geddes, L.A. and Baker, L.E. *Principles of Applied Biomedical Instrumentation.* New York: John Wiley & Sons, 1968.

23. Geddes, L.A., Tacker, W.A., and Cabler, P. A new electrical hazard associated with the electrocautery. *Med Instrum.* 9:112–13, 1975.

24. Gessner, U. Vascular input impedance. Edited by D.H. Bergel. In *Cardiovascular Fluid Dynamics,* Vol. I, pp. 315–49. New York: Academic Press Inc., 1972.

25. Goldstein, S. and Killip, T., III. Comparison of direct and indirect arterial pressures in aortic regurgitation. *N Engl J Med* 267:1121–24, 1962.

26. Gothert, M. and Wendt, J. Inhibition of adrenal medullary catecholamine secretion by enflurane. *Anesthesiology.* 46:400–403, 1977.

27. Green, J.F., Fitzwater, J.E., and Clemmer, T.P. Septic endocarditis and indwelling pulmonary artery catheters. *JAMA.* 233:891–92, 1975.

28. Guyton, A.C. Regulation of cardiac output. *Anesthesiology.* 29:314–26, 1968.

29. Guyton, A.C. *Textbook of Medical Physiology,* 4th ed. Philadelphia: W.B. Saunders Co., 1971.

30. Hamilton, W.F. and Dow, P. An experimental study of the standing waves in the pulse propagated through the aorta. *Am J Physiol.* 125:48–59, 1939.

31. Hansen, A.T. Pressure measurement in the human organism. *Acta Physiol Scand.* Supplement 68, 1949.

32. Herrick, J.F. Measurement of blood flow. (Guest editorial) *Med Instrum.* 11:134–35, 1977.

33. Higgins, M.V. and Dzubay, D. Transducer-associated bacteremia. North Carolina. *Morbidity and Mortality Weekly Report* 24:295, 1975. Altanta: Center for Disease Control.

34. NFPA No. 76C: *High-Frequency Electricity in Health Care Facilities,* 1975. Boston: National Fire Protection Association, 1975.

35. Hurzeler, P., DeCaprio, V., and Furman, S. Endocardial electrograms and pacemaker sensing. *Med Instrum.* 10:178–82, 1976.

36. Johnstone, R.E. and Greenhow, D.E. Catheterization of the dorsalis pedis artery. *Anesthesiology.* 39:654–55, 1973.

37. Kanai, H., Iizuka, M., and Sakamoto, K. Problems in the measurement of blood pressure by catheter insertion, abstracted. 8th International Conf. on Medical and Biological Engineering. Chicago, 1969.

38. Krucoff, D., Reed, P.C., Moss, G.S., and Siegel, D.C. Catheter-manometer dynamic response improvement, abstracted. *JAAMI.* 5:126, 1971.

39. Lappas, D. et al. Indirect measurement of left atrial pressure in surgical patients. Pulmonary capillary wedge and pulmonary artery diastolic pressures compared with left atrial pressure. *Anesthesiology.* 38:394–97, 1973.

40. Lappas, D.G., Powell, W.M.J., Jr., and Daggett, W.M. Cardiac dysfunction in the perioperative period: pathophysiology, diagnosis, and treatment. *Anesthesiology.* 47:117–37, 1977.

41. Lenfant, C. Medical devices control: a panacea? (Editorial) *N Engl J Med.* 289: 1310, 1973.

42. Leonard, E., Hajdu, S. Action of electrolytes and drugs on the contractile mechanism of the cardiac muscle cell. Edited by W.F. Hamilton, and P. Dow. In *Handbook of Physiology, Section 2, Circulation.* Vol. I, pp. 151–98. American Physiological Society. Baltimore. The Williams and Wilkins Co., 1963.

43. Lowenstein, E., Little, J.W., and Lo, H.H. Prevention of cerebral embolization from flushing radial artery cannulas. *N Engl J Med.* 285:1414–16, 1971.

44. Maki, D.G., Weise, C.E., and Sarafin, H.W. A simiquantitative culture method for identifying intravenous catheter-related infection. *N Engl J Med.* 296:1305–09, 1977.

45. Malt, R.A. The thoughtful appendectomist. (Editorial) *N Engl J Med.* 275:962, 1966.

46. McCutcheon, E.P., Baker, D.W., and Wiederhielm. Frequency spectrum changes of Korotkoff sounds with muffling. *Med Res Eng.* 8:30–33, 1969.

47. McCutcheon, E.P., Evans, J.M. and Stanifer, R.R. Direct blood pressure measurement: gadgets versus progress. *Anesth Analg.* 51:746–58, 1972.

48. McNeil, K. and Minihan, E. Medical technology regulation and organizational changes in hospitals. Presented at the American Sociological Association meeting. New York, September 3, 1976. Revised and published as: Regulation of medical devices and organizational behavior in hospitals. *Adm Sc Q.* 22:475–90, 1977.

49. Milnor, W.R., Bergel, D.H., and Bargainer, J.D. Hydraulic power associated with pulmonary blood flow and its relation to heart rate. *Circ Res.* 19:467–80, 1966.

50. Milnor, W.R. Pulsatile blood flow. Physiology in Medicine. *N Engl J Med.* 287:27–34, 1972.

51. Orwell, G. *Animal Farm.* New York: Harcourt, Brace and Company, 1946.

52. Pace, N.L. A critique of flow-directed pulmonary arterial catheterization. *Anesthesiology.* 47:455–65, 1977.

53. Pascarelli, E.F. and Bertrand, C.A. Comparison of blood pressures in the arms and legs. *N Engl J Med.* 270:693–98, 1964.

54. Peterson, L.H. The dynamics of pulsatile blood flow. *Circ Res.* 2:127–39, 1954.

55. Raftery, E.B., Green, H.L., and Gregory, I.C. Disturbances of heart rhythm produced by 50 Hz leakage currents in dogs. *Cardiovasc Res.* 9:256–62, 1975.

56. Remington, J.W. The physiology of the aorta and major arteries. Edited by W.F. Hamilton and P. Dow. In *Handbook of Physiology, Section 2, Circulation.* Vol. II, pp. 799–838. American Physiological Society. Baltimore: The Williams and Wilkins Co., 1963.

57. Robin, E.D. Of seals and mitochondria. *N Engl J Med.* 275:646-52, 1966.

58. Roy, R., Powers, S.R., Jr., Feustel, P.J., and Dutton, R.E. Pulmonary wedge catheterization during positive end-expiratory pressure ventilation in the dog. *Anesthesiology.* 46:385-90, 1977.

59. Sawyer, P.N., Ramsey, W., Stanczewski, B. et al. A comparative study of several polymers for use as intravenous catheters. *Med Instrumen.* 11:221-30, 1977.

60. Schoenberg, A.A. Couvillon, L.A., Baker, C.D., and Toronto, A.F. Standard for electrocardiographic devices. (Fourth Draft, January 20, 1977.) Developed under FDA contract with Utah Biomedical Test Laboratory, University of Utah Research Institute. Salt Lake City.

61. Scholander, P.F. The master switch of life. *Sci Am.* 209:92-106, 1963.

62. Shin, B., McAslan, T.C., and Ayella, R.J. Problems with measurement using the Swan-Ganz catheter. *Anesthesiology.* 43:474-76, 1975.

63. Sonnenblick, E.H. and Skelton, C.L. Oxygen consumption of the heart: physiological principles and clinical implications. *Mod Concepts Cardiovasc Dis.* 40:9-16, 1971.

64. Sonnenblick, E.H. and Strobeck, J.E. Current concepts in cardiology: derived indexes of ventricular and myocardial function. *N Engl J Med.* 296:978-82, 1977.

65. Spencer, M.P. and Denison, A.B., Jr. Pulsatile flow in the vascular system. Edited by W.F. Hamilton and P. Dow. In *Handbook of Physiology, Section 2, Circulation.* Vol. II, pp. 839-64. American Physiological Society. Baltimore: The Williams and Wilkins Co., 1963.

66. Stamm, W.E., Colella, J.J., Anderson, R.L., and Dixon, R.E. Indwelling arterial catheters as a source of nosocomical bacteremia. An outbreak caused by flavobacterium species. *N Engl J Med.* 292:1099-1102, 1975.

67. Stegall, H.F. A simple, inexpensive, sinusoidal pressure generator. *J Appl Physiol.* 22:59-92, 1967.

68. Strandness, D.E., Jr. and Sumner, D.S. *Hemodynamics for Surgeons.* New York: Grune & Stratton, 1975.

69. Swan, H.J.C., Ganz, W., Forrester, J. et al. Catheterization of the heart in man with use of a flow-directed balloon-tipped catheter. *N Engl J Med.* 283:447-51, 1970.

70. Van Bergen, F.H., Weatherhead, D.S., Treolar, A.E. et al. Comparison of indirect and direct methods of measuring arterial blood pressure. *Circulation.* 10:481–90, 1954.

71. Wallace, C.T., Carpenter, F.A., Evins, S.C. and Mahaffey, J.E. Acute pseudohypertensive crisis. *Anesthesiology.* 43:588–89, 1975.

72. Wang, H.H., Liu, L.M.P. and Katz, R.L. A comparison of the cardiovascular effects of sodium nitroprusside and trimethaphan. *Anesthesiology.* 46:40–48, 1977.

73. Weinstein, R.A., Stamm, W.E., Kramer, L., and Corey, L. Pressure monitoring devices: overlooked source of nosocomial infection. *JAMA,* 236:936–38, 1976.

74. Whitcher, C. Blood pressure measurement. Edited by J.W. Bellville and C.S. Weaver. In *Techniques in Clinical Physiology (A Survey of Measurement in Anesthesiology).* Toronto: The Macmillan Company, 1969.

75. Wiggers, C.J. The circulation and circulation research in perspective. Edited by W.F. Hamilton and P. Dow. In *Handbook of Physiology, Section 2, Circulation.* Vol. I, pp. 1–10. American Physiological Society. Baltomore: The Williams and Wilkins Co., 1963.

76. Yanof, H.M., Rosen, A.L., McDonald, N.M., and McDonald, D.A. A critical study of the response of manometers to forced oscillations. *Phys Med Biol* 8:407–22, 1963.

77. Yanof, H.M. *Biomedical Electronics.* Philadelphia: F.A. Davis Co., 1965.